# *Praise for* Come Hither

"I think of Dr. Gloria Brame as the Dr. Albert Einstein of kink. She explores and researches the world of SM and BD with great intellect, heart, and sensitivity. Just as $E=MC^2$, Gloria + erotically gifted + excellent writing skills = the not so square book, *Come Hither*. Brame makes the world a sexier and delightfully kinkier place!"

> —Annie Sprinkle, kinky porn star, educator, internationally acclaimed artist, and author of *Annie Sprinkle: Post Porn Modernist*

"Dr. Brame has given us a sorely-needed Baedeker to the secret land of SM."

> —Graham Masterton, author of *The Seven Secrets of Really Great Sex*

"Dr. Gloria G. Brame is simply the best tour guide I know for your travel in the world of kinky sex."

> —Robert T. McIlvenna, M.Div., Ph.D., President, The Institute for Advanced Study of Human Sexuality

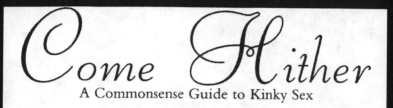

# Come Hither
## A Commonsense Guide to Kinky Sex

## Dr. Gloria G. Brame

A Fireside Book
Published by Simon & Schuster
New York  London  Sydney

FIRESIDE
Rockefeller Center
1230 Avenue of the Americas
New York, NY 10020

FIRESIDE and colophon are registered trademarks
of Simon & Schuster, Inc.

Designed by Diane Stevenson

Manufactured in the United States of America

10   9   8   7

Library of Congress Cataloging-in-Publication Data
Brame, Gloria G.
    Come hither : a commonsense guide to kinky sex / Gloria
G. Brame.
        p. cm.
    Includes index.
    1. Sex.  2. Sexual fantasies.  3. Sexual deviation.  I. Title.
  HQ23.B835  2000
306.7—dc21
                                                        99-049475

ISBN  978-0-684-85462-5

# Contents

**CHAPTER TEN:**

## Power Relationships

**CHAPTER ELEVEN:**

## The View from the Top: Sexual Dominants

**CHAPTER TWELVE:**

## The View from the Bottom: Sexual Submissives

# Come Hither

# CHAPTER ONE

# Introductory Kink

## KINKY CONFESSIONAL

Nine years ago, I began working on a book called *Different Loving: The World of Sexual Dominance and Submission.* When my coauthors and I started out, we assumed we would be researching the small sexual subculture of dominance and submission (also known as B&D and SM) to which we belonged. Basically, we sought to write a book *about* people like us *for* people like us—people who knew what they liked but felt they needed to understand more about kinky sex from a broad perspective.

On this assumption, we researched the history and practice of SM, and directed all our interview efforts at people in the "Scene" (a nickname for the kinky subculture in the United States). Aiming for diversity, we talked to as many different kinky people as possible—gay, straight, transgendered, bisexual. We recruited them from kinky newsgroups on the Internet, sometimes according to their fetishes; we wrote letters to SM/fetish organizations and attended club events, distributing flyers; and we asked friends to tell friends about our book project.

In the end, we had hundreds of terrific interviews, covering not only an amazing spectrum of sexual variations, but spanning a diverse range of religions, ages, races, and social classes. There was, however, one serious limitation on the sample: All of the people we interviewed knew they were kinky and had decided, at some point in their lives, to join the SM subculture to one degree or another.

In fact, the number of people who actually find their way into the Scene represents only a small fraction of the total number of American adults who enjoy erotic variations that would be classed, clinically, as sadomasochistic or fetishistic. During the course of our research, that larger group revealed itself to us. It comprised a largely conventional, completely in-the-closet, and clinically unacknowledged segment of society that neither seeks out kinky contacts nor even admits to having kinky fantasies to anyone other than a life-partner—or possibly a professional dominatrix.

My husband, Will Brame (who was my coauthor on *Different Loving*, along with Jon Jacobs), and I were at first bemused when, at conservative literary gatherings, we would be deluged by people who asked us lurid questions. At one such prim gathering where the women wore Birkenstocks and the men wore colorless ties, one thirty-something repeatedly squealed loudly in disgust as we talked about our research. Later, she approached us privately. Dreading yet another onslaught, we were taken aback when she asked us this question: Her ex-boyfriend liked her to pee on him before sex. Would we consider this kinky?

Well, yes. We would. It's certainly kinky enough for there to be a clinical term for it (*urophilia,* or a love of urine).

The squealer was only the first of an unfathomable number of ordinary, conservative people we've met since who similarly react first with horror, then fascination, when we describe our work.

The most curious confessions came from a media coach. She told us later that she had been worrying all day that we would show up in biker jackets, with chains around our necks and piercings everywhere else. Our business suits apparently comforted her because by the time our meeting was over, she had confided that while she was shocked by the people who "threw their waste on one another" (which is how she characterized the squealer's boyfriend's fetish), she could easily understand why people would enjoy being infantilized (put into diapers and treated like babies). She spoke quite fondly of the Elia Kazan movie *Babydoll,* in which a grown woman sleeps in a crib and sucks her thumb. In fact, the coach talked quite a long time about both fetishes, and with strong emotion too.

What was really going on in her mind? Why was peeing on someone else more morally reprehensible than dressing in a diaper and peeing oneself? Is this some rule of sexual etiquette my parents never taught me: You can pee on yourself, but not on your friends?

Once the book came out, the confessions reached a fever

pitch. It seemed that every place we went, there was always one person, and usually more, who wanted to tell us their secrets. On one book tour, a Washington reporter confided that he had a foot fetish; a Southern bookstore manager whispered a throaty tale about the time his girlfriend begged to be his "loveslave"; a California radio personality admitted to us that his ex-wife liked him to slap her face during sex; and so on. Occasionally, people blocked our path, grabbed our elbows, hurriedly blurted out a sexual confession, and then darted away before we had time to react. Hit-and-run confessors, as it were.

Where did they all come from? How many of them (or us) are really out there? At present, there are no hard data on how many adults engage in consensual kinky sex of one type or another. Sex theorists have made estimates ranging from 5 to 50 percent of the adult population, with the consensus opinion closer to 10 to 15 percent. From my own experiences, I know the interest is much higher than the consensus.

In 1987, under the handle "Angelique," I founded an SM educational outreach/support group on Compuserve. The group was part of a larger network of specialized sexuality support groups in Compuserve's Human Sexuality Forum (HSX). At the time, the HSX Forum had roughly 50,000 subscribers. When we set up the new SM group, we expected only a tiny membership. This was partly because other support groups already were in place for certain fetishes and partly because we required members to fill out an online application stating that they had a personal interest in SM/fetish sexuality. Even though people could apply under pseudonyms, we believed this requirement would help to filter out gawkers.

In three months, our membership swelled from an initial sign-up of a few dozen people to over 3,000. By the second year of operation, we had drawn over 15,000 people to our membership roster and were hosting the single busiest message board on HSX.

The advent of the Internet has been an eye-opener. For the first time, kinky people from around the world—whether living in rural communities in the United States or major cities in the Third World—had free access to materials that confirmed there are others just like them out there. And access them they did!

By 1994, the alt.sex.bondage newsgroup on UseNet (since abandoned) was attracting nearly half a million visitors every week. Dozens of smaller newsgroups, for more specialized fetish interests, were springing up left and right, as were IRC chat-rooms devoted to BDSM. By the following year, dozens of kinky sites had set up shop on the World Wide Web, offering everything from amateur photos to personal diaries and educational resources.

In 1996, I built gloria-brame.com and continued the work of *Different Loving*. One of my Web site's most popular features is the "Kink Links Catalogue" (http://gloria-brame.com/love8.htm), a resource guide to over 1,500 SM/fetish Web sites. As of mid-1998, according to my research, there were roughly 3,000-plus sites catering to SM/fetish interests. My site alone draws roughly 2,000 people daily from places as far away as Peru, Bahrain, and Singapore.

Needless to say, I get a ton of E-mail. Most fall into two categories: people asking to be listed in my links catalogue and people requesting personal advice.

The queries about listings are interesting for two reasons. First, there are so many of them! Second, while I expected to see lots of bondage, spanking, cross-dressing, and infantilist sites, until the requests began pouring in I had had no idea, for example, that there are enough people sexually aroused by toy balloons (yes, the kind you blow up at kiddy parties) to support the hundred or so sites which now cater exclusively to that fetish.

The personal letters fall roughly into two camps. One is made up of pleas for advice from people who, until discovering kink on the Internet, believed themselves the only ones in the world with these interests. When they read other people's writings about subjects they've never permitted themselves to talk about, it has an immediate and powerful effect. They are both thrilled and desperately frustrated by the discovery because they don't know how or where to begin.

The second type of personal letter comes from people who know there are others like themselves but who have not been able to find a sympathetic partner. Reduced to pursuing their interests in secret, surfing the Web or anonymously subscribing to kinky publications that are sent in plain brown wrappers to discreet postal drops, they often feel trapped in troubled marriages to spouses who angrily reject their sexual needs. Their attempts at communicating their needs or introducing variations in bed have resulted in fights and tears. Some blame their partners for being puritanical; others blame themselves for being sinful or sick. Yet almost all hope that I can give them advice to help save their relationship.

This book will provide answers for them, as well as their partners, their friends, family members, healing professionals, and anyone else dealing with kinky sex issues. Even if you've never tried kink, and don't intend to try it, this book will round out your personal understanding of the range of acceptable sexual variations that consenting adults may enjoy. Frankly, in an age when STDs make many of us choose safe-sex alternatives to intercourse, and when we're all living longer and remaining sexually active longer, picking up new ideas on ways to spice up your erotic life may not be such a bad idea.

I'll guide you through all the key issues related to kinky sex, beginning with the most basic questions (What is normal sex? Are there others like me?). I'll tackle more advanced topics as well, including how to hang on to a relationship when one partner can't accept the other's kinks; religious and moral conflicts about sexual differences; and how to differentiate between a positive, loving kinky relationship and an abusive one.

Drawing on the thousands of letters from the broad mix of people who have written me these past eight years, I will use representative questions to start discussions of a vast range of fascinating facts about kinky sex. I'll explore what kinky sex is (and what it isn't), how to talk about it with your loved ones, how to deal with your own shame or embarrassment about your fantasies, and how kink is incorporated into stable, loving relationships.

Along the way, there will be tons of practical advice, including lists (such as "Clamps, Cuffs, and Crosses," a guide to the wide range of kinky adult toys, with notes on how they are used); entertaining and revealing quizzes you can take alone (or with your friends); and some purely humorous excursions. I've even developed a special primer for you: "Speaking the Kinky

Lingo" (in the appendix, on page 307) is a glossary of common slang used in the kinky communities. Use the glossary whenever you come across an unfamiliar kinky word or expression—it'll be there.

Now, before launching into the dos and don'ts and hows and whys of kinky sex, I want to prepare you for topics that may alarm you, facts that may surprise you, opinions that may upset you, and sexual scenarios that may excite you. So let's start with what I consider to be a fundamental document for anyone who wants to bring a truly open mind to these issues.

Reprinted below are the "Basic Sexual Rights," a ten-point list approved by the Ethics Committee of the Fifth World Congress of Sexology.* This document takes the enlightened view that sexual rights are a basic part of our human and civil rights, as granted by the U.S. Constitution.

After each numbered "right," I will add my own explanatory comments so you understand exactly what each one means.

## BASIC SEXUAL RIGHTS

1. The freedom of any sexual thought, fantasy, or desire.

   Everyone is entitled to his or her private thoughts, no matter how bizarre they may seem to someone else.

2. The right to sexual entertainment, freely available in the marketplace, including sexually explicit materials dealing with the full range of sexual behavior.

   If you want to watch pornography, read smutty magazines, or patronize sex-workers (strippers, prostitutes, etc.), you can do so without stigma.

3. The right not to be exposed to sexual material or behavior.

---

*The Complete Guide to Safe Sex by the Senior Faculty of the Institute for Advanced Study of Human Sexuality, ed. Ted McIlvenna, M.Div., Ph.D. (Beverly Hills, Calif.: PreVenT Group/Specific Press, 1987): pp. x–xi.

If you do *not* want to be exposed to pornography or sex-workers, you should not be forced to come in contact with them.

4. The right to sexual self-determination.

This means you may do as you wish with your body, sexually speaking. You can be celibate if you choose; you can sleep around; you may masturbate or you may abstain from all gratification. In other words, it is up to you to make the choices that feel morally right for you, without persecution from others.

5. The right to seek out and engage in consensual sexual activity.

This means you can sleep with consenting partners.

6. The right to engage in sexual acts or activities of any kind whatsoever, providing they do not involve nonconsensual acts, violence, constraint, coercion, or fraud.

All types of sex are acceptable as long as both people involved give their informed mutual consent. Using force or lying to get sex is wrong.

7. The right to be free of persecution, condemnation, discrimination, or social intervention in private sexual behavior.

Gays, lesbians, sadomasochists, fetishists, swingers, transgenderists, bisexuals, polyamorists, and all other sexual minorities should be free to pursue their sexual needs without being hassled or shut out of society.

8. The recognition by society that every person, partnered or unpartnered, has the right to the pursuit of a satisfying consensual sociosexual life free from political, legal, or religious interference and that there need to be mechanisms in society where the opportunities of sociosexual activities are available to the following: disabled persons; chronically ill persons; those incarcerated in prisons, hospitals, or institutions; those disadvantaged because of age, lack of physical attractiveness, or lack of social skills; the poor and the lonely.

Every adult, no matter their abilities or age, or their social or health status, is entitled to the comfort and pleasure of sexual contact with a consenting partner.

9. The basic right of all persons who are sexually dysfunctional to have available nonjudgmental sexual healthcare.

People with sexual problems are entitled to sympathetic counseling.

10. The right to control conception.

It's up to each individual to decide whether they wish to use birth control.

Did you find these sexual rights controversial? Whatever your own feelings about the list of rights, I hope you will think them over. They lay the groundwork for you to see beyond the misconceptions and prejudices that our culture imposes on us all. If you can accept, for example, that every human being is entitled to his own thoughts, no matter how strange, and that some of those thoughts are likely to be sexual, then it will not be a big leap for you to accept that everyone has a right to have strange sexual thoughts.

In this book, all sexual behaviors that occur by consent among mentally competent adults are seen as acceptable, valid, and normal expressions of adult sexuality.

You may not approve of them, you may not want to act on them, but being able to accept that they are a normal phenomenon, and not something to fear, is a great first step. That's why I describe them as acceptable sexual variations. I use "acceptable" instead of "right" or "wrong," "sick" or "healthy," because those terms all carry moral or medical judgments.

I'll leave moral doctrine to spiritual leaders. As a sexologist, my point of view is that a kind of sex is right when it feels good to the adults having it and wrong when it creates upset and unhappiness. Meanwhile, classifying sexual behaviors as diseases is a concept that has long outlived its usefulness, except as ways for lawyers to get clients acquitted and for quacks to profit by falsely promising cures.

I believe sexual behaviors should be viewed the same way we view all human behaviors. Some sexual behaviors—rape, for example—are criminal, because they are acts of violence against a victim. Some are pathological (e.g., compulsive self-mutilation) and generally indicate a much larger mental disorder (such as schizophrenia). But, by far, the majority of sexual behaviors are neither.

Now I'd like you to consider "The Five Fallacies of Kinky Sex." It addresses the biggest misconceptions about kink, so we can get those out of the way right up front.


## THE FIVE FALLACIES OF KINKY SEX

### 1. Kinkiness Can Be Cured

FALSE.

There is no scientific evidence of any kind that people can be cured of their kinks.

The fact is that attempts at cures have universally failed. Those who offer to cure someone's sexual nature generally do more harm than good. Some clients report feeling emotionally devastated, others betrayed, because they were given false hope. Some blame themselves for the failure and feel even guiltier than before.

Distressingly few helping or medical professionals receive adequate training in sex issues. Only a small handful of graduate programs even offer comprehensive curricula on sex. So, although they may be sincere and persuasive, people who offer cures are just as misinformed as the people who come to them.

At best, they may teach you to hate your own needs (through aversion therapy, where you learn to associate hateful things with the things that turn you on) or to sublimate your desires. But bottling up sexual feelings or punishing yourself for having them does not cure you of those feelings. Instead, it usually creates deeper conflicts.

Competent sex counselors do not advertise cures. Instead, they work with clients to find morally acceptable, socially responsible, and emotionally positive ways of dealing with their clients' sexual identity.

## 2. Perversions Are Caused by Trauma in Childhood

FALSE.

Despite the strides we've made in some areas of the medical sciences, there has been little forward progress in sexuality research. To date, there has been neither organic nor genetic proof to explain fetishes or sadomasochism. Nor is there any proof that childhood traumas produce the same results in different people or that trauma must always be present for someone to grow up with a love of pain or a fetish for high heels.

The soundest theory, basically unchanged since the late nineteenth century, is that our sexual identities are formed through a combination of genetic predisposition (meaning that our DNA comes encoded with sexual quirks) and life experiences. In other words, the best guess is that nature and nurture combine to shape our sexual identity.

Recent advances in genetic research open the door to finally finding out whether body chemistry or brain structure can explain things such as homosexuality or transgenderism; perhaps, one day, it will reveal facts about sadomasochism and fetishism too. I also hope there will be more studies on the cause-and-effect relationships between early childhood development and sexual orientation. But for now, all data are inconclusive.

## 3. People with Kinky Desires Have Psychological Problems

A TRICK FALLACY!

The answers to this are true and false.

First: False. There is no proof that people with unusual sexual fetishes or desires are any less functional than other people. Instead, there is considerable evidence that, as a group, kinky people are in the mainstream: stable, middle-class family people who maintain careers and participate in their communities. In other words, they are socially functional, which is a standard of psychological normalcy.

Second: True. People with sexual kinks do tend to seek out

counseling. But one must consider why they do. Generally, it's because their feelings conflict with the feelings they are told they should have. For example, if the world tells you the most sexually appealing part of a woman's body is her breasts, and you find breasts boring but feet to be an instant turn-on, you are going to feel confused. If someone you love rejects you because of it, you're going to feel even worse.

Like anyone else, a kinky person doesn't want to feel as if she or he is alone in the world. No one wants to be rejected; no one wants to feel unlovable. In the face of the criticism kinky people face from families and lovers, often on a daily basis, it is not suprising that they turn to professionals for support.

## 4. Kinky People Can't Form Good Relationships

FALSE.

As noted above, kinky people do tend to seek out counseling, particularly when they are having conflicts with partners about their sexual needs. But sex and relationship problems are what motivates most people to go into therapy. The difference is that when "vanilla" (non-kinky or straight) relationships fail, people accept it as a common problem of modern life. When kinky relationships fail, however, people automatically assume that the blame rests on the partner with unusual sexual desires.

But as Mom always said, "It takes two to tango." In other words, it's a question of compatibility. Kinky people are bad partners with people who cannot accept their kinks (or have other incompatabilities). Otherwise, they are as likely as anyone else to form lasting, committed relationships.

## 5. Kinky People Can't Get Aroused by "Regular" Sex

FALSE.

Not only can they get aroused by it, many of them never have anything *but* regular sex.

Although we tend to think of kinky people as the leatherclad denizens of underground clubs, most people who are aroused by kinky things never have contact with that world. For any one of a number of reasons (social position, career, marital status, children, religious beliefs), they remain closeted, enjoying ordinary, productive sex lives with straight partners—even though they may fantasize about their fetishes during sex.

Millions more adults regularly indulge in bondage, spanking, role-play, and so on as foreplay. For them, these are erotic games that add spice to monogamous relationships, extend the arousal period, and enhance orgasms.

There are indeed fetishists who are only aroused when the object of their fetish is present, and hard-core SMers who have little or no interest in intercourse. However, the vast majority of kinky couples include oral, anal, or vaginal sex as a regular part of their intimacy.

# CHAPTER TWO

# What's Your Kink Quotient?

## KNOW THY KINKY SELF

Now that you've tackled the basics, you need to put kinky things into proper perspective: It's time to learn something about yourself. So get a paper and pen handy.

You've heard of IQ tests. How about a quiz that rates your kinkiness? The Kink Quotient Quiz will help you (and your partner) understand more about your sexual identity. Though some of the questions below are lighthearted, your answers will add up to a clear picture of your attitudes towards sexual variety. Find out if you're a "kink genius"—someone who has more fetishes than an anthropological museum—or see if you are "kink challenged"—the kind of person who looks at a paddle and actually thinks of kayaking.

Select the answer that best reflects the way you think. Burn your answer sheet afterwards if you must, but be honest. Then follow the scoring guide below.

### Using the Quiz as a Communications Tool

You can use this quiz as a tool to open up dialogue about sexual issues with friends and partners. Just make sure that, in addition to pen and paper, you also bring the right attitude: This quiz is a frank but playful way to learn more about each other's sexual attitudes, not a competition or an opportunity to sneak in a few criticisms or lob any china.

## Couples

If you're doing this as a couple, take turns reading the questions and the answer choices aloud, then write your answers down privately. When you've gone through all twenty questions, exchange sheets and score each other's answers.

Now comes the hard part: the truth! Have your partner read aloud your score and the description below that matches it, and you do the same. Then go back and review the quiz together, question by question. Before moving to the next question, take turns explaining to one another why you chose your answers.

## Groups

If you're really brave, try this as a game next time you have a party. Pick a leader, who distributes score sheets and then reads the questions and answer choices aloud. After the players have filled out their score sheets, have each one write his or her name in the upper-right-hand corner, then fold the corner down twice and either clip, tape, or staple the sheet so the name can't be seen.

The leader will collect these sheets and put them in a hat or basket, then pass it around until each player has removed a sheet to score. The leader will then read the scoring guide aloud, so everyone knows how many points to give each question.

Finally, taking turns, everyone should read the total score on the sheet he or she drew, and the others can take turns guessing which sheet was filled out by whom. The person who correctly identifies the most "kink geniuses," "happy hedonists," and "kink challenged" is the winner.

At which point the winner should get a prize spanking.

# The Kink Quotient Quiz

MULTIPLE CHOICE: Select a, b, or c.

1. The chances of me experimenting with anything beyond heterosexual intercourse are:

   a. Pretty good, especially when it comes to things like mutual masturbation or using adult toys.
   b. What!? People are still having heterosexual intercourse?
   c. Dim, slim, and nonexistent.

2. When my lover starts to talk about his (or her) "equipment," my first thought is that he (or she) is referring to:

   a. Genitals.
   b. Handcuffs.
   c. Computer hardware.

3. I've often said, "Size does not matter!" Privately, though, I think size really does matter when it comes to:

   a. Genitals.
   b. Bondage racks.
   c. Video monitors.

4. When I come across an ad that uses SM and kinky imagery to sell a product, my instant reaction is to:

   a. Giggle or gawk at it.
   b. Feel titillated and perhaps even turned on.
   c. Wonder what the world is coming to and feel sad.

5. I think that all the tattoos, piercings, bondage, and other kinky images in the music videos on MTV are:

   a. Wild and crazy, but not in a bad way.
   b. Pale imitations or distortions of the real thing.
   c. Ridiculous at best and often downright disgusting.

6. If my partner asked me to do spanking or bondage, I would:

   a. Probably try it at least once to please my partner.
   b. Ask, "Your toys or mine?"

c. End the relationship or insist my partner seek counseling.

7. I can understand why someone might experiment with light bondage, but when it comes to whips and pain:

   a. That's too weird for me.
   b. I understand it even better.
   c. I think it's all sick.

8. Some people get turned on by wearing saddles and acting like ponies. My first question is:

   a. How do you kiss someone with a bit in his mouth?
   b. Can they recommend a good tack shop?
   c. Are they getting help for their problem?

9. My attitude on public nudity could be summed up as follows:

   a. It can be a very liberating experience.
   b. I prefer people to be dressed—in slave-collars and chastity belts.
   c. If God had intended us to be naked, He would have . . . oh, wait a minute! No, seriously, I believe nudity should be reserved for private moments.

10. In my perfect sexual world, people would:

    a. Do whatever they want, as long as it doesn't involve pain.
    b. Do whatever they want, as long as they are adults who are doing it by mutual consent.
    c. Respect the rules set out by society or religion.

TRUE, FALSE, OR SOMEWHERE IN THE MIDDLE: Answer true or false or "somewhere in the middle" to the following ten questions.

11. I have never done anything that could qualify as "kinky."

TRUE _____     SOMEWHERE IN THE MIDDLE _____     FALSE _____

12. I've never fantasized about bondage, forced sex, spanking, or anything else that could be considered kinky

TRUE _____     SOMEWHERE IN THE MIDDLE _____     FALSE _____

13. "Sexual variations" is just a nice term for perversions. Whether it's homosexuality or kink or anything else, it's morally wrong and people need to stop doing it.

TRUE _____     SOMEWHERE IN THE MIDDLE _____     FALSE _____

14. I've never noticed that I have a particular erotic interest in a fetish object (feet, high heels, boots, leather, rubber, underwear, cigars/cigarettes, body hair, etc.).

TRUE _____     SOMEWHERE IN THE MIDDLE _____     FALSE _____

15. Porn movies, graphic magazines, erotica, and all other explicit sexual material turn me off.

TRUE _____     SOMEWHERE IN THE MIDDLE _____     FALSE _____

16. Using "adult toys" is unnatural; it may even be wrong.

TRUE _____     SOMEWHERE IN THE MIDDLE _____     FALSE _____

17. Sexual experimentation can get out of hand. People shouldn't open that can of worms.

TRUE _____     SOMEWHERE IN THE MIDDLE _____     FALSE _____

18. It's okay if a man is dominant in the bedroom, but it's wrong for a woman to take that role.

TRUE _____    SOMEWHERE IN THE MIDDLE _____    FALSE _____

19. Religious, philosophical, or political beliefs are more important than an individual's sexual desires.

TRUE _____    SOMEWHERE IN THE MIDDLE _____    FALSE _____

20. I'll never regret it if I don't experiment with kinky sex.

TRUE _____    SOMEWHERE IN THE MIDDLE _____    FALSE _____

## SCORING

MULTIPLE CHOICE:

Every "a" answer = 5 points.

Every "b" answer = 10 points.

Every "c" answer = 0 points.

TRUE/FALSE/SOMEWHERE IN THE MIDDLE:

Every "true" answer                               = 0 points.

Every "somewhere in the middle" answer   = 5 points.

Every "false" answer                              = 10 points.

## 150–200 POINTS: KINK GENIUS

If you've scored at the very high end of this range, you are probably already immersed in a BDSM lifestyle. Even if you've never shared your kinks with anyone but your life-partner, you have few inhibitions when it comes to sexual experimentation. You place personal sexual happiness above what you perceive as playing by other people's rules. For this reason, you don't judge others for whatever it is that turns them on.

You see yourself as an enlightened, progressive individual for whom a varied erotic life is an essential ingredient of personal happiness. You like to read about sex of all kinds, and enjoy erotica and pornography. Even if you don't share or understand a particular turn-on, you're willing to try it if the circumstances (or partners) are right.

In purely clinical terms, and according to the standards established by the American Psychiatric Association, you would be classified (depending on your specific interests) as either a fetishist or a sadomasochist.

## 100–150 POINTS: HAPPY HEDONIST

You have a positive, accepting attitude towards sex and keep an open mind about what others do, whether or not you fully understand their choices. When you discover that people close to you are sexually unusual, you accept them as they are and may even enjoy talking to them in depth about what turns them on.

For the most part, you love sexual variety and get a thrill from trying new erotic twists. You tend to be attracted to sexual adventurers who, like you, embrace a range of sexual opportunities. In addition to BDSM acts, you may also be interested in bisexuality, swinging, group sex, triads (threesomes), and other unconventional erotic liaisons.

Under the right circumstances, and with the right partner, you may experiment, particularly with sensual sexual dominance and submission, light bondage or spankings, and role-play ("naughty nurse" or "naughty schoolboy" scenarios, for example). You might even have a mild fetish or two (for example, you may be turned on by sensuous foot massages or seeing your partner in black leather).

## 50–100 POINTS: STRAIGHT BUT NOT ENTIRELY NARROW

For the most part, you sincerely believe that intercourse between members of the opposite sex is the only really normal sex act. Although you may also engage in oral or anal sex, or mutual masturbation, that's as far as you want to go, and even those acts seem a little edgy to you.

Probably you were raised with fairly conservative attitudes about proper sexual conduct. You aren't entirely sure that sex is something people should discuss anywhere but behind bedroom doors, and even there it is not an easy subject for you to talk about.

Still, generally speaking, you are are open-minded enough to believe that how consenting adults choose to conduct their sex lives is really no one's business but their own. You may not entirely approve of them, you probably don't want to hear about them, and you may not choose to socialize with them, but you don't wish them harm.

## 0–50 POINTS: KINK CHALLENGED

Oh, dear. Yes, I'm afraid so. You are Kink Challenged. But cheer up—you probably don't mind. Not only isn't kink your cup of java, you'd rather perish of thirst than sip that brew

Your qualms about kinky sex are the results of your social training. Chances are you were raised in a strict environment where sex education mainly consisted of warnings about the sinfulness of lust, and punishments for behaviors your elders didn't like (such as masturbation, premarital sex, etc.). Your adult inhibitions may extend to oral sex and any other kind of contact that is driven by an instinct for pleasure instead of an urge to reproduce. More than a few of you are not entirely comfortable with heterosexual intercourse with your spouse.

Even if you secretly have kinky thoughts, you feel that people who act on such feelings are asking for trouble. You believe that perversion inevitably leads to disaster. When you hear news stories about brutal crimes that involve SM-type activities, you feel justified in your beliefs. You would never knowingly enter into a relationship with someone you knew to be perverted, unless they vowed to change.

On the high end of this score, you probably disapprove of kinky people and wish they would change or somehow vanish. At the low end of the scoring scale, you may actually feel they are evil or insane.

However, you are reading this book, which suggests there may be some curiosity on your part or possibly some secret doubts about your sexual identity. Or perhaps someone you know has asked you to read it. Whatever your reasons, something is going on in your life that prompts you to look for answers.

It's possible that your attitudes are not in balance with the realities of your life right now. If you find yourself overcome by intense negative emotions as you read through this book, it's more than possible that your sexual identity is a source of great trouble and distress for you. This inner turmoil may account for your feelings of anger or disgust when you see others acting in ways you'd never permit yourself to act.

Quite often, it is true that we hate most what we fear most. It may be time for you to take a closer look at your attitudes and how they have developed over the course of your life. Before moving on to the rest of the book, take a little time to reflect again on both the questions and your answers. If you took the test again, would you answer all the questions in exactly the same way?

## Some Questions for Couples to Ponder

Did you and your partner have similar scores? In what areas did you seem to have the biggest differences? Were you surprised by how you scored? Were you surprised by your partner's score? What, if anything, did you learn from this exercise?

# CHAPTER THREE

# The Kink in All of Us

*I'm a thirty-four-year-old woman and I've been married for eight years. My husband and I have a good sex life, or so I thought until recently when he asked me to tie him up and spank him before we have sex. I know it's trendy now to talk about outrageous sex, but I always thought things like that were sick. Am I being a prude? What is normal sex?*

## WHAT'S NORMAL?

The plain truth is that we don't know what "normal" sex is, at least not in the sense of what is natural for people to do in bed. We don't know how we might behave if we were not pressured to conform to social and religious standards. Since we can't raise children in a vacuum, we can't study humans scientifically to see what kind of sex would be normal if we followed only our imaginations and biological urges.

Instead, scientists can only study and speculate. In February 1999, the *Journal of the American Medical Association (JAMA)* published results from the most significant study of sexual dysfunction since the Kinsey Report (published in 1948). Over 3,000 participants (1,749 women and 1,410 men) between the ages of eighteen to fifty-nine were interviewed. Scientists were stunned to learn that over 40 percent of the women and 30 percent of the men were "sexually dysfunctional," which was defined as not wanting to have sex on a regular basis, having difficulty getting sexually aroused, or being unable to achieve orgasms.

Put another way: If you were in a room with twenty people (ten women and ten men), seven of them would be clinically classified as sexually dysfunctional. That's something to think about at the next company picnic.

The data published by *JAMA* suggest that it's normal (or very,

very common) to be sexually dysfunctional. Is it possible, perhaps, that many of the terms we use to classify sexual behavior (such as "sexual dysfunction," "abnormal sex," and "perversion") merely express prudish and moralistic attitudes towards sex, and not a realistic, science-based understanding of the true diversity of human sexual identity? What if all this "dysfunction" is not so much a lack of interest in sex but a lack of interest in the type of sex that society considers normal? It seems like good common sense to me that if 40 percent of any group can't get turned on by what they're doing, they ought to consider doing something else.

Some fascinating insights into human sexual behavior come not from research on humans but from research on our closest biological relative, the bonobo. To this primate, sex is a form of socializing and an outlet for energies that might otherwise turn violent. He is a hot-blooded hedonist who has sex of all kinds—intercourse, oral sex, masturbation—with partners of both sexes and all ages. In human terms, the bonobo is a promiscuous, bisexual swinger. And talk about kinky! The female bonobo beats up males who refuse to satisfy her sexually.

Left to our own imaginations, would people be as creative? Observations of the world around us suggest that we already are. But organized society depends on people controlling their sex drives, so it is our social and religious institutions that have taken on the burden of establishing standards for us to live by.

Most conventional institutions define normal sex as reproductive sex, or sex intended to create new life—in other words, missionary-position sex between man and wife. Depending on your faith, and where you live, anything outside that narrow definition may be condemned as sinful or prosecuted as illegal.

The reproductive standard helps religions and societies maintain a certain order and, equally important, gives them some measure of control over population growth. But this standard does not recognize sex as a healthy, natural, and even necessary expression of the life force within us.

Sex—meaning consenting sex between loving partners—is good for us. It creates vital bonds of intimacy, relieves stress, gives us emotional fulfillment, and generally helps us to maintain a state of mental equilibrium. It also feels wonderful.

But given the contradiction between the conventional standard of "normal" and the feelings and desires we were born with, many people feel desperately confused about sex. Even though they may do it for the pleasure it brings, they often feel ashamed for failing to live up to the standards imposed by their churches and communities.

Confusing matters even more is the fact that standards of what's normal vary from generation to generation and place to place. Some sexual behaviors we condemn today were considered quite acceptable in different times and different places. In centuries past, churches sanctioned marriages between adult males and young girls. Nowadays, a man who woos an underaged girl is considered a pedophile, and would quickly end up in jail—or at least on Jerry Springer.

Once upon a time, not so very long ago, men who forced rough kisses on women or who otherwise pressured women into sex were perceived as macho men with enviable testosterone levels. Nowadays, we perceive them as date rapists. And the women who once were scorned and blamed for "inciting" men's lust by letting themselves be coerced into sex are now considered victims.

Similarly, in the Victorian era, polite society maintained that sex for women was nothing more than a nauseatingly unpleasant duty, something a proper lady did with her eyes closed. In the 1990s, a woman who is so disgusted by intercourse that she can only endure it with her eyes closed would be urged to get psychological help.

The list goes on and on. In different places, at different periods in human history, you can find societies that accepted (and even encouraged) homosexuality, prostitution, pedophilia, polygamy, and incest. In other places, at other times, sexual behaviors we now consider harmless—such as masturbation or looking at naughty pictures—were viewed as moral and spiritual abominations that threatened the fiber of society.

So standards change.

Now let's talk about erotic thrills such as bondage, spanking, and rough sex and see where they fit into the big picture of human sexuality.

Dr. Alfred Kinsey, whose pioneering work on human sexual behaviors remains the most comprehensive, estimated that as many as 50 percent of all adults may experiment with some type of rough or painful play during sex. (This would include things like biting, squeezing, pinching, and digging nails into your lover's flesh.) Most contemporary sexologists agree that about 10 to 15 percent of the adult population regularly engages in kinky sex of one kind or another. Respected authority and *Joy of Sex* author Alex Comfort has even advocated bondage as a way for couples to increase sexual pleasure and intensify orgasms.

The *Diagnostics and Statistics Manual* of the American Psychiatric Association, in its current fourth edition, asserts that kinky sex is a problem or disorder *only* when it impairs a person's social adjustment or ability to have intimate relationships. If a kinky person can function normally in society, his sexual orientation or preferences alone do not make him a candidate for treatment.

One of the most interesting documents I've seen on sexual minorities is, oddly enough, an official report prepared by the Central Intelligence Agency. The publication "Sexual Behaviour and Security Risk: Background Information for Security Personnel" (October 1993, Richards J. Heuer, Jr.) reports that transgendered and kinky people are not necessarily any more or less likely to be security risks than so-called sexually normal ones. In his executive summary, author Heuer writes: "Self-control, social maturity, strength of character, and overall psychological adjustment are more important security indicators than the specific sexual practices in which people engage." Perhaps what is most interesting about this document is that we seldom think of the CIA as a source of enlightened opinions on kinky sex.

Throughout history, hundreds of millions of people have regularly and safely engaged in sexual variations that nineteenth-century scholars and scientists labeled as perversions. You can find instructions in the Kama Sutra on how to slap your lover to drive her to liquid passion. In ancient Greece, rich old men kept handsome young boys as erotic playmates as a kind of status symbol. Cross-dressers played a role in the belief systems of several Native American cultures. In medieval Europe, Joan of Arc dressed and lived as a man in order to follow her spiritual destiny. Other practices—such as flagellation (whipping), sexual bondage, the use of sex aids (such as dildos), and virtually everything else you might have thought are new phenomena have been known and documented throughout history.

Of course, we hear far more today than we did fifty years ago about homosexuality, cross-dressing, fetishism, and other allegedly abnormal sexual interests. This is not because people today are kinkier than their ancestors. It's safe to assume that our great-great-grandparents and those who came before them harbored all the same kinds of feelings we have.

What has changed in our times is that our media have become so sophisticated that we are deluged with information about the world—and among that information is, inevitably, information about diverse sexual practices. The fact is, there is a huge public thirst for any and all kinds of information about sex, which only encourages the media to pursue those stories even more (as the Monica Lewinsky/President Clinton scandal all too amply demonstrated).

The background statistics for my Web site show that people from literally every country in the world (or at least every one that has Internet access) visit weekly. I've received thousands of letters from people who had just realized that there were other people out there who shared their secret fantasies. Whether they hailed from Cairo, Illinois, or Cairo, Egypt, Paris, Texas, or Paris, France, they write more or less the same thing: that until they logged onto the Net, they thought they were the only ones who needed different types of erotic experiences to feel sexually complete.

From my point of view, "normal sex" simply means sex that consenting adults enjoy fantasizing about and doing. Since the facts demonstrate that lots of people enjoy kinky sex, then kinky sex falls well within the range of normal human behavior. If your partner wants to be tied up or spanked, then this is what is normal for him, and he can find millions of other people who would agree with him that bondage and discipline are good clean erotic fun.

But there are two partners here. Self-determination is a basic sexual right for you both. If you are fearful or unhappy about experimenting, if sexual variations turn you off, for whatever reason, then what's normal for him may just not be acceptable for you. If so, it is *your* right to say no.

My advice is that you stop worrying about "What is normal?" and instead ask yourself the only really important question: "What is acceptable to me?"

## ARE YOU READY TO EXPLORE?

*I'm forty-seven. Ever since I was a boy I have had these fantasies but I never had the courage to do anything about them. I live in a conservative town and I have a career I need to protect. I can't tell anyone who knows me what I'm into. They'd want to lock me away. But the older I get, the harder I'm struggling with these needs. I'm afraid that if I don't do something about them, I might die feeling like I never lived. Do you have any advice for me? I don't know if I'm really ready, but I feel like time's slipping away.*

One of the most painful decisions for most people is determining not only when they should start experimenting with kink, but if they should experiment at all. There are any number of reasons why most people with kinky fantasies never act on them. Typically, people worry most that people close to them— relatives, friends, coworkers—will find out and ostracize them or, worse, force them to seek psychiatric help or report them to legal authorities.

Some of these risks are quite real. If you live in a small, conservative town where population size or your career make you a highly visible member of the community, you run a genuine risk of being snubbed should people discover that you like to crawl around in front of cruel women and lick their boots. Why, I can't say, but apparently some people have a problem with that.

There are legal risks as well. Some local laws prohibit the sale or purchase of BDSM smut; different states vary considerably in their attitudes towards kinky sex. While it is unlikely ever to occur, legally speaking, an adult who gives his or her partner an erotic spanking could—should local authorities choose to do so—prosecute the spanker on charges of battery. As a general rule, there is no distinction between criminal battery and an erotic spanking or whipping in the eyes of the law.

Still, the primary reason most people do not act on their fantasies has less to do with social disgrace or legal jeopardy and more to do with inner conflict about their sexual identities. They may repress and deny their feelings, particularly if they believe the world around them condemns the very things that turn them on. An intense antipathy or hostility to an unusual form of sex may, in fact, indicate that the person is in denial about his or her own needs and desires.

One of the most interesting scientific studies in recent times was conducted in 1996 at the University of Georgia. In "Is Homophobia Associated with Homosexual Arousal?" (H. E. Adams, L. W. Wright, and B. A. Lohr, *Journal of Abnormal Psychology* 105[2], 440–45), scholarly researchers reported on the results of a study of homophobia.

The researchers wired up two male study groups. The first group consisted of thirty-five homophobic men and the other consisted of twenty-nine non-homophobic men. Using "penile plethysmography," a medical technique that measures erections, the study revealed that the group of men who had previously expressed the most deep-seated hatred or dislike of homosexuality were far more likely to be aroused by gay pornography than the second group.

In other words, the ones who "hated" gays were most turned on by gay sex. The data are as follows: 54 percent of the first group were definitely aroused, 26 percent were mildly aroused, and 20 percent of the men were not aroused at all. In the second (non-homophobic) group, 24 percent were definitely aroused, 10 percent were mildly aroused, and 66 percent of these men were not aroused at all.

The data allow room for speculation about other types of unconventional sex, including kinky sex. As the University of Georgia study suggests, those who express outward hostility towards sexual differences may be struggling with their own desires for these things.

Another reason people may refrain from acting on their desires is that they fear that if they should ever give in to their kinky desires, they will become addicted to them and ruin their lives.

Most adults have sexual fantasies that, on occasion, stray into pretty wild territory. Threesomes, foursomes, and moresomes; hanging off chandeliers or dancing naked on the beach; and hundreds of other fanciful adventures we never admit out loud. Sex studies have shown that rape fantasies are very common too. But while our imaginations may fly uncontrollably over such extreme fantasies, sane people deliberately draw a line between fantasy and reality, and leave their most extreme fantasies as fantasies only.

This applies directly to BDSM and fetish fantasies as well. There is so much fear built up around kinky sex that some genuinely believe that BDSM is a swirling vortex of sin that will suck a person in helplessly. (My goodness, that almost sounds sexy.) The fact is that kinky sex, between consenting adults, is just good (albeit unusual) sex. It is no more or less dangerous than other kinds of sex—which means that it *is* dangerous when the partners are troubled or destructive, and it is lovely when the partners are moral and good to one another.

Below is a quiz that will help you to figure out whether you should consider exploring your kinky fantasies. After you've scored yourself, you will see my comments on where you stand, kink-wise. I am not basing my analysis on your social situation or your religious beliefs, but on how large a role kink already plays in your imagination.

Before you pick up your pencil, a final comment: Sometimes we think we're giving 100 percent truthful answers; then, after our minds open just a bit wider and absorb new information and ideas, we realize we might have answered some questions differently.

As you continue reading this book, you'll see which letters and sections you identify with most, and will gain new insights. Periodically, you may want to take some of the tests in this book over again to see whether you score the same way.

Use this quiz as a guide in your journey towards a fuller understanding of your own sexual identity, then take it again when you finish reading the book. Your second set of scores, in all likelihood, will more accurately reflect your true feelings.

## "Ready . . . or Not?" Quiz

Answer true or false to each of these ten simple questions. At the end, you will find a scoring guide.

1. I've had kinky fantasies ever since I was a child.

TRUE _____     FALSE _____

2. Kinky fantasies have sometimes obsessed me to the point where I can't stop thinking about them for hours or days at a time.

TRUE _____     FALSE _____

3. At different times in my life, I have secretly acted out my kinky fantasies just to relieve the tension (or lust) they stir.

TRUE _____     FALSE _____

4. I spend a lot of time or money on toys, clothes, or pornography related to my fantasies.

TRUE _____     FALSE _____

5. I have enacted kinky/fetishistic fantasies with partners.

TRUE _____     FALSE _____

6. My most sexually passionate relations have been with partners who did kinky things with me (even though we may never have admitted out loud it was kinky).

TRUE _____     FALSE _____

7. When I've been intimate with a conventional sex partner, I've felt that something was missing somehow.

TRUE _____     FALSE _____

8. Even when I'm really enjoying regular sex, my mind wanders to SM/fetish fantasies because they get me even more excited.

TRUE _____ FALSE _____

9. I always have kinky fantasies when I masturbate.

TRUE _____ FALSE _____

10. The best (or only) way for me to achieve climax is to visualize kinky images at the moment of orgasm.

TRUE _____ FALSE _____

## SCORING GUIDE
Give yourself 10 points for every "true" and 0 for every "false."

## 60–100 POINTS: EMPHATICALLY READY

You already know, or should know, that your kinkiness is a part of you that will not go away. Most likely, it's the missing ingredient that has made a conventional sex life lackluster or has created intimacy problems for you. If you scored at the high end (90–100) yet have only been in vanilla relationships, those relationships have probably been unstable or have felt like uphill battles, filled with power struggles.

Obviously, you still have many choices ahead about how to act on your desires in safe and moral ways, but to deny this very real part of yourself can only lead to further personal unhappiness.

The fact is that if you've carried these feelings with you for most of your life, if you spend a great amount of time thinking about them, and if your natural inclination in bed is to conjure up kinky images, you will not find fulfillment until you give yourself permission to translate your fantasies into reality.

If you scored 80–100 and have never acted on your impulses, then you may be emotionally harming yourself by repressing a fundamental part of your God-given nature. This can only add to the overall stress in your life. Among other problems, sexual repression causes guilt, shame, depression, feelings of isolation, addictive behaviors, self-hatred, rage, violence, anxiety, and eating disorders.

So you are ready. Very ready. The next question is whether you're ready to be ready. I never push people to do things they don't want or need to do. But if you know in your heart that you do want and need these things, then I encourage you to accept yourself as you are and to seek out positive, healthy ways to express the kinky (but still wonderful) you.

In upcoming chapters, I'll give you plenty of advice and information on exploring your needs.

## 20–50 POINTS: READY, BUT NOT NECESSARILY RARING TO GO

You are "kink possible"—someone who harbors a few sexual quirks and has a fertile sexual imagination. However, the desire to incorporate kink into your life isn't a driving need for you. Under the right circumstances, and with the right partner, you might be as kinky as the wildest of us. But you are unlikely to suffer any serious emotional strife if you don't pursue it. You could thrive in a vanilla relationship.

You may, however, be interested in expanding the boundaries of pleasure. You probably have a few cherished sexual fantasies that you would like to realize with a willing partner. You may crave a thrill-of-a-lifetime, one-time experience. Or you may enjoy "bedroom kink": kinky sex that is primarily used as foreplay, and that doesn't extend into a daily relationship—the way, for example, master/slave relationships or transgenderism continue into people's daily lives.

Whichever applies, you will not suffer any ill consequences if you don't experiment. Yes, you could stand to gain, especially if you have a wholesome, uninhibited attitude towards trying new things in bed. Acting out some special, particularly hot scenarios might deepen your intimacy with partners, and could even improve your performance in bed, possibly giving you and your partner better orgasms. But these are "maybes." If you have other issues surrounding kinky sex—for example, religious or social inhibitions—the negatives could outweigh the positives for you.

My advice is to wait until you find the right person and the right opportunity, rather than to run out and begin exploring.

Let it enter your life naturally, in the course of an intimate relationship. This is especially true if you scored at the low end of this range (30–40).

## 0–20 POINTS: HOLD IT RIGHT THERE

Kink is not a missing ingredient in your life. If anything, it may be a source of conflict in your relationship if your partner requests kinky sex. You are completely satisfied with conventional sex and your ideal partner feels the same way.

It's still possible that you've had a kinky fantasy or two in your life, or that you've peeked at some naughty magazines; you may even have occasionally masturbated about something weird or acted out a partner's fantasy at his or her request. But these experiences are common to us all and don't make you kinky— just sexually curious and imaginative.

Just as I try not to push people into doing things they aren't ready for, I also don't like to push people away from trying things they think could be fun. If you want to see whether kink is your cup of tea, that is your choice. But don't be disappointed if it isn't as exciting in reality as it seemed in fantasies or if you are left wondering, afterwards, what all the fuss is about.

If you've scored in this category, the only really good reason for you to explore kink is if your partner scored in a different one. Experimenting with kink may not significantly enhance your own sexual satisfaction, but it could make your beloved much happier. For some couples, that is all the reason they need to explore new territory together.

### JUST SAY MAYBE

*My girlfriend has confessed she wants to be my sex slave. I agreed at first but then she told me she wants me to whip her. I loved the idea of being her "master" in bed, but there is no way I will hit a woman. I really care about her, and I don't want to go back on my word, but I can't go that far. I'm afraid if I tell her the truth I'll lose her but that if I play along I'll end up somewhere I don't want to go.*

It is a simple, albeit painful, fact of life that your "no" could mean that your partner will ultimately look for someone who can give her what she needs in bed. If you think your partner "isn't like that," think again. People who clearly express an intense sexual need know what they want and are serious about finding it. This is as true of women as it is of men. So, if you care about hanging on to your partner, it is in your best interest to work with her towards a compromise solution that keeps your relationship on solid ground.

The most important thing you can do is to open an honest dialogue about sexual limits. See if you can find a comfortable middle ground between her "Yes, yes, please, yes!" and your "No way, Jose!" A satisfying compromise can be the cement that bonds you for the long haul.

On page 45 is a list of eight talking points couples can use to begin such a dialogue. The goals of these talking points are to help you listen to one another and to better understand each other's attitudes about kinky sex. Teamwork and mutual understanding are foundations for a fulfilling sexual relationship, kinky or otherwise.

First, make a date to have your conversation. Don't spring it on your partner or issue it as a challenge. Instead, plan to be together in as relaxed an environment as possible—over milk and cookies in the kitchen, or cozied up on the living-room couch with soft music in the background.

When you start, flip a coin to see who goes first. The first person will answer all eight questions sequentially. Then switch roles and have the second person answer them while the first one listens quietly.

Watch for body language. Is he shrinking away or folding his arms tightly? If so, this topic is making him tense. Is she looking at you nervously for reactions or prompts? Chances are she feels insecure and is worried that you will think less of her if she gives the "wrong" answer. These body movements are part of the picture of your lover's attitude towards the subject—often, such signals are more revealing than what a person says.

Whatever you do, try not to judge or criticize. It's possible your partner may give some answers that are illogical. That's fine. Sexual feelings aren't logical; they are emotional and often irrational. The key here is to listen and learn more about your partner's limits and desires, and then to work from there by seeing how much each of you can accommodate the other without giving up the excitement you each deserve.

## EIGHT TALKING POINTS ON KINKY SEX

1. Do you remember any particular message about sex (good or bad) that came through to you when you were growing up?

2. What's the difference to you between "regular" sex and "kinky" sex? Where would you draw the line between the two?

3. Is it confusing or upsetting to find out that there is no black-and-white definition of "normal" sex?

4. What do you think about specific aspects of kink, like bondage, spankings, cross-dressing, fetishes, etc.? Are any of them "better" than others?

5. If someone you respect and trust (a therapist, a clergyman, a parent) reassured you that these things were all normal, would that give you "permission" to try them?

6. What is your biggest reason for fearing or disliking kinky sex? (Or, conversely, what is the big turn-on to you?)

7. If you knew that your partner could not be happy without a kind of sex you don't really understand, would you experiment with it for your partner's sake?

8. Whose sexual satisfaction is most important to you: your partner's or your own? Or are both equally important to you?

After you've both answered all eight questions, you have two options. You may simply stop at this point and make a date to have a follow-up conversation. There is a value in postponing the discussion of your answers. This will give you a cooling-off period to think about what each of you said and to think of some key points you'd like to raise next time.

The second option is to have the conversation right away, when your answers are still fresh in your mind.

Whatever you do, make sure to cover some basic ground. First, explore how your opinions and experiences differed. What were some of the biggest surprises for each of you when listening to the other's answers?

If either of you repeatedly express negative feelings about kink, and have little or no interest in a compromise, for whatever reason, you probably will need professional or peer counseling to make progress. If, on the other hand, some of your answers overlapped, you can begin working from there. For example, let's say you want bondage and pain, while your partner refuses to experiment with pain but has no problem with bondage. You can compromise, at least for now, by doing bondage together and seeing how that goes.

Is it everything you want?

No.

But is something better than nothing?

What do you think?

Personally, I think it's a step in the right direction. If the bondage experiences are fun for you both, the level of trust—and, one hopes, sexual excitement—between you will grow. This kind of positive reinforcement may empower you to expand your erotic repertoire into new areas over time.

Although these are talking points, and not a test, you can score yourselves. If you fight, you lose. If you get through the entire dialogue without tears or recriminations, you win.

## WHEN YOUR PARTNER IS HOSTILE

For those of you whose partners express anger or hostility about your kinks, here is a one-question pop quiz to try.

# Dr. Brame's One-Question Wonder Quiz

**Question:** *If you could change any of the following things about your partner, what would it be?*

his/her salary level

his/her career

his/her spending habits

his/her weight

his/her drinking or smoking

the amount of time he/she spends with you

his/her behavior towards relatives (including your children)

his/her friends

his/her hobbies

his/her personal habits

his/her sexual fetish

anything else

On a piece of paper, list each of the above (earnings, spending habits, weight, etc.) and then rank them in descending order. The one that bothers you the most should be number one, and so on.

Now look at each other's list. Where does the kinky sex fall? Is it in the number one place on the non-kinky partner's list? If it is, go over the list together and question your partner—is kinky sex really more of an issue to him or her than *all* of these other typical lovers' complaints?

If your partner feels this is so, you may be dealing with a bigger problem that you thought. Your sexuality has become a prime focus of your partner's rage and frustration. The question is, "Why?" Does the hostility stem from an early trauma in your partner's life? Is your partner feeling conflicted between the lessons of childhood and the realities of adulthood? Or have you provoked the anger through inappropriate or aggressive demands?

Whatever the problem, it must be dealt with in order for you to have a healthy sex life. Professional counseling is recommended to help resolve the sexual conflicts.

That's the bad news. The good news is that almost all of you will find that the kink falls further down the list of complaints. This is more typical and will help put your unusual needs into a realistic perspective. For one, you can point to the list and show your partner that you have better things to fight about. This may sound funny, but fights about sex go straight to the heart of a relationship and can undermine its stability.

Sexual quarrels never end at the bedroom door, either. If your partner targets your sexual quirks as the cause of all the strife in your relationship, he or she will begin to interpret everything you do through a filter of suspicion and negativity. ("The only reason he's being nice to me is because he wants me to do that weird thing with him in bed!")

If other issues are more important, it's possible the fights about the kinky sex are actually not about sex at all. A sexual quirk is an easy target. "If only she didn't want me to hit her, everything would be just fine!" This feeling is common but naive. It may be emotionally safer for your partner to attack your fetish than to grapple with more complex problems, particularly ones for which he or she may have to accept some blame.

If this is the case—that the fights about sex are your partner's way of venting frustration about other issues in your relationship—you would do well to identify the real cause and work on it, either alone or with the help of a counselor, before trying to move ahead with your requests for kinky sex.

*I've been trying to get my wife to go along with my fetish for rubber ever since we got married five years ago. I've left magazines around, hoping she'll get the hint. I tried talking to her once but we ended up fighting. I know it's weird, but this is me and I just can't wait any more. Last week I ordered a rubber suit from a fetish catalogue. I am planning to get dressed up one night before she comes to bed and then surprise her. What do you think?*

Even I, polymorphous pervert that I am, would find it a tad disconcerting to open my bedroom door and find Diver Dan waiting in full rubber regalia. But the real problem with your plan is that it involves deception. Coercing or tricking someone into kinky sex is a moral line no consenting adult should cross. It doesn't matter if you're asking to be done or asking to do: Respect for your partner's right to self-determination is the first step towards reaching a loving arrangement.

Believe me, I do understand the intense urge to act on a sexual impulse *right this very minute*. We all have it, and the clinical term for it is "horniness." But if you haven't been able to convince your partner to indulge one of your fetishes or kinks, shock tactics are not the solution. Instead, you might send your true love screaming from the room, possibly all the way back to her mother's house.

Foisting one's fetish on a partner, whether she likes it or not, tells her that you are in this for yourself and yourself alone. If talking with your partner doesn't seem to lead anywhere, and you want to try action instead, you have a much better option. My advice is to keep your rubber suit in the box and to follow this short self-guide to kinky romance.

## Step One: Slay Your Personal Demons

One of the major reasons people fail to successfully introduce their partners to the joys of kinky sex is because they themselves are so conflicted that that they project a negative attitude right from the start. Instead of discussing their desires candidly, they use coy, manipulative techniques that send a clear message that they are ashamed.

Plainly put, you won't convince someone that kink is fun if you secretly worry that it's sick. When reluctant or inhibited partners sense your shame, it reinforces their belief that such desires are evil or wrong. The worst thing you can do is to bring your conflicted feelings about kinky sex to someone even more conflicted than you. That's just looking for trouble.

So, for example, leaving little clues around the house in hopes your lover gets the idea is futile unless he or she already shares the interest. You aren't going to convert anyone by showing them magazines or books. They may be sexy to you, but she's not seeing them through your eyes. She comes to them with all her own inhibitions, limits, and opinions in place. If she found them distasteful before, discovering a lurid magazine leering at her from the linen closet will only upset her even more.

Don't play games or dump your negative attitudes on partners and then expect them to be eager to experiment. It won't happen. Work on your own issues first. Read books on the subject, join support groups, participate in Internet discussions, or seek counseling with a competent professional. Wait until you feel more at peace with yourself and can present your needs in a calm, sensible manner.

## Step Two: Be Clear About Your Erotic Goal

Are you seeking a one-time experience to spice things up? Or are you hoping that this will become a regular part of your intimate life? Many partners who are open enough to try something once or twice feel angry or betrayed when they find out that their lovers expect it all the time.

I've known all too many couples in which the women went along with their partners' kinks until they were married or had children, at which point the women insisted on throwing away the sex toys and acting "more like adults." In most of these cases, the women claim their initial willingness to be kinky was part of their youthful experimentations with sex, and not something they committed to doing forever.

This is a sad situation. An opportunity was lost. Someone who enjoys kink at twenty should be able to enjoy it at forty, sixty, and eighty. So what happened? Although I've heard men say they were "tricked" into marriage by women who were happy to do kinky things until the papers were signed, my guess is that at some point their partners felt betrayed and decided to withhold kinky sex as punishment. The betrayal may not have had anything to do with the kink itself. Withholding sex from one's partner is perhaps humanity's oldest form of interpersonal mental torture.

It's also possible that your partner was always ambivalent about having kinky sex but was afraid to admit it to you in the early stages of the relationship, for fear that you would reject him or her. Although this is unfortunate, it is a very human weakness to pretend to be something we aren't in order to impress someone else, particularly someone we want to marry.

Before you lay all the blame on your partner, look into your own heart. Were you completely honest about what you wanted? Did you downplay your own interest in kink? Or did you make your partner feel that you're more interested in your fetish than her?

Chances are that if you take a cold, hard look at your relationship you'll see that both partners have contributed to the problems that face you now. But there is no time like the present to work on improving your sexual rapport.

If kink is a fixed aspect of your fantasy life, and something you need consistently, your partner needs to know. After all, if you've made a commitment to spend your lives together, you must love one another for who you are, and not for who you think the other should be. It won't be easy to talk about such intimate, revealing subjects. Still, it is far easier to discuss them in private now, in hopes that you can reach an agreement of some kind, than to publicly fight over them in divorce court later, when all hope for compromise is gone.

If you would be happy with only occasional indulgences, make sure your partner understands that too. Someone who might be averse to doing kink all the time may well be game enough for an occasional walk on the wild side.

Finally, if you are already married or have children together, know that it is never too late to renegotiate the terms of your relationship. Predicate your conversation with your partner on your commitment to staying in the relationship but make it clear that just as each of you, as individuals, has evolved over the years, so have your sexual needs. Discuss these changes and let him or her know where you stand today and where you hope to go in the future.

Again, if you've come to the conclusion that kinky sex is what you need to be satisfied, your partner needs to know and has the *right* to know. Only through open communication will you be able to reach a viable solution.

## Step Three: Let Them Know They Turn You On

I recently heard from a nice gentleman who was anxious to find some way to convince his wife to let him kiss and make love to her feet. She refused, then asked him whether this meant that he thought her feet were the only attractive part of her body.

He was surprised when I told him that it sounded like his wife felt insecure about her looks. All he had heard was her rejection. It took him a few minutes to realize that his wife, who he then admitted felt insecure about her body size, may have feared that he was focusing on her feet because he didn't like the rest of her—something that was simply untrue.

When a lover suddenly introduces an unusual request, the partner's defenses may immediately kick into high gear. A woman who thinks her breasts are too small may believe that the real reason you spend so much time nibbling her toes is because you agree with her. Similarly, a man who's worried about his penis size may be troubled if you seem more interested in his backside than his front side.

The best way to deal with such insecurities, should they arise, is to reassure your partner that you love him or her in totality, but that certain body parts just naturally turn you on more than others. You can explain that while other people may find the female breast to be the most erotic part of a woman's body, you think that her (fill in the blank: belly button, fingernails, tush, hair) is/are wondrously sensuous. You can explain, also, that being able to unite your love for the whole person with your fetish for particular parts of his or her body is a peak experience for you, both emotionally and erotically. And emphasize that adding such variations to your sex life together only makes your partner's already adorable self seem even sexier and more adorable to you.

You might also encourage your partner to confide in you which parts of your body he or she finds sexiest. Your mate might just surprise you by revealing that there are a few spots on your body he or she secretly finds oddly appealing. If you can turn this into a little lover's game—"I'll show you my favorite spots if you show me yours"—all the better. There is nothing like gentle humor in bed to make a difficult topic easier to explore.

## Step Four: Pamper Your Way to Success

Another reason people find it difficult to convince their partners to experiment with variant types of sex-play is, quite simply, because the partner doesn't see what he or she will get out of it.

While you may be lucky enough to be involved with a saint whose love for you is so unselfish that just pleasing you is enough, most of us are ordinary human beings who don't find it terribly thrilling to be fantasy facilitators. If your partner doesn't share your enthusiasm, he may even feel that you are only "using" him to get your jollies.

I frequently get letters from people who are so intent on getting their partners to try something that they seem to forget that their partners have needs too. If you are in this boat, it's time to start rowing. The golden rule applies: If you want to be done unto, it's time for you to learn how to do.

Use your imagination. Other than intercourse, what could you do for your partner to put him or her "in the mood"? Does he like back rubs? Do candlelight and roses make her sigh softly? Have you ever taken a bath together, and embraced while tenderly soaping each other?

Or maybe you'd set your lover afire if you just agreed to do the dinner dishes once in a while.

Whatever the inducement, buttering up your beloved with sensual treats is both shrewd and seductive. The working mom who sees your request for kink as just another demand on her overstressed life might be more receptive if the payoff includes pampering of a type she enjoys. The straight-arrow man in your life might feel much more kindly towards tying you up and teasing you for an hour if he knows it will end in a superb blow job.

The key here is finding those turn-ons or loving gestures that let your partners know that their satisfaction is as important to you as your own. They may not share your fascination for spike heels or leather jockstraps; on the other hand, letting you kiss said apparel might not seem as onerous if you also do something that puts a smile on their face and an orgasm in their loins.

In the chapters ahead, I'll talk in depth about specific types of scenarios you can play out to help encourage your partner in the right direction.

**FLUFFY STUFF**

Purely for fun, and to help ease some of the tension these discussions may cause, try sharing this bit of fluffy stuff with your lover.

### Five Ways That Kinky Sex Is Like Music

1. It's a creative art.

2. Practice makes perfect.

3. Every Good Boy Does Fine.

4. The larger your repertoire, the more exciting your performances.

5. You can move to the beat (ouch!).

### HOW I LEARNED TO STOP WORRYING AND LOVE THE WHIP

About fourteen years ago, when I was first coming to terms with the fact that I was a sexual sadomasochist, I visited an SM club and saw a man take a vigorous whipping from a leather-clad dominatrix. I wasn't shocked because, after all, it was an SM club, and this was what SM was supposed to be about. But I was disturbed by the sight of a man, right there in front of me, groaning and writhing as welts rose on his back.

At that point, my experimentation had been limited to such things as light spankings, gentle bondage, role-play, and sexual teasing. I'd used crops, but I'd never hit anyone hard enough to leave marks. The whipping I saw was a whole other level of intensity and one, I thought as I watched, I would never reach.

Still, I was fascinated and, in retrospect, probably aroused. When they were done, I approached them cautiously. They turned out to be a very friendly, sweet couple from New Jersey. He was an architect; she was his office manager. No longer in their sadist/masochist roles, their humanity came through loud and clear.

They told me, beaming with happiness, that after years of living together, they had just formally announced their engagement. The public whipping was a kind of betrothal ceremony. They had planned it out for some time, at his request, and it symbolized her acceptance of him as her husband, and slave, for life.

It was an awakening when I grasped that what I'd just witnessed—and completely misjudged as brutal and cold—was, in fact, a pact between lovers. She wore his ring and he wore her welts. I don't know who felt prouder. Though I couldn't entirely understand the welts at the time, I did understand, instinctively, that these two people had done something wildly passionate to celebrate their love. What could be more romantic?

This experience came back to me when I began work on *Different Loving*. I knew I'd be writing about a number of fetishes and perversions that did not turn me on. At the same time, the book took a sympathetic approach towards kink, and relied greatly on extensive interviews with people who enjoyed all these things. To represent them fairly, I needed to understand how they felt. I needed to know, from the inside, why this or that particular fetish was so erotic. So, in my own mind, I looked for a hook, for some element of their kinks that connected to my own. Though it took some time and thought, little by little, I began to get it.

For example, I initially had some difficulty understanding foot fetishism. It didn't trouble me, but I just didn't understand why some people found feet to be so erotic. Until then, I'd never paid particular attention to a lover's feet. But then I began thinking . . . well, why *not*? There's no law that says a behind or a chest is sexy but that feet are not. Like a lot of women, I'd always found men's hands to be sexy; I love men's chests and shoulders too, and also their nipples, their thighs, their necks. So why not their feet?

I began to see the feet as merely another extension of the beloved. Besides, a well-shaped foot can be aesthetically pleasing (Michelangelo certainly put as much work into sculpting the feet of David as he did the other parts). Toes have a big cuteness factor—plus, people wiggle them when they're having fun. I also grasped the symbolism of foot worship: Kissing a foot is an act of humility and obedience. Traditionally, the foot (particularly in a boot) is a symbol of brute power. To lie prostrate at someone's feet is an ultimate act of servility.

Although fetishists are drawn to feet for many different reasons, for me it was these three aspects—accepting every part of the human body as lovely, the cuteness factor of toes, and the power relationship implicit in foot worship—that resonated with my erotic personality. Ultimately, I saw how strange it was that I had previously drawn an invisible mental line around a man's knees, or that I had felt uneasy when a lover showed a fetishistic zeal for my feet.

I can't say that understanding these fetishes significantly changed my own basic likes and dislikes. But once I was able to make the emotional connection between what turned me on and what turned others on, once I let go of some of my own inhibitions and one-sided views, I could take the next step: I could learn to eroticize a partner's turn-on and enhance the pleasure for us both.

With a partner who has an intense erotic response to feet, I can now find many different ways to give him the experience he is seeking while getting what I like from the experience too. For example, I rather enjoy being kissed and treated like a queen— and what could be more queenly than having someone humbly kiss my feet? I like a clear power dynamic—when someone kneels at my feet, it enhances my feelings of being in command. And, being the playful type, I've found that tickling a man's feet when he is in bondage elicits some astonishing sounds.

I guess you could say that I've made a lot of strides in the foot department.

I feel strongly that all couples who are sincerely interested in enhancing their mutual erotic pleasure can achieve similar results if they too find some common ground to build on. Even if you maintain different perspectives on *why* something is sexy, you can still enjoy it together. Think of it this way: You and your partner might both agree you like a particular movie, yet each of you could like it for different reasons. The same goes for sex: We all get something slightly different out of what we do in bed, anyway. You can make those differences work for you instead of against you.

In "How to Eroticize Anything," below, you will learn techniques to help expand your erotic horizons. But first, please remember two things.

First, inhibitions are normal. They are not always bad, either. Don't feel obligated to throw away all your inhibitions (and don't drink alcohol or take drugs to help you get rid of them, either). Take it all one step at a time, trying new things only when and if they feel good to you.

Second, if you have serious reservations about doing something, don't do it. It's that simple. Better to say no when you can than to wake up the morning after with regrets.

The bottom line: Don't set the impossible task of trying to eroticize things that genuinely leave you cold. The point of the guide below is to help you expand your erotic horizons. It is not intended to coax you to do things that offend, frighten, or otherwise upset you.


## HOW TO EROTICIZE ANYTHING

### 1. Relax

The first and most important step is to get comfortable with the fetish or kink your partner wants you to try. The best way to do this is to educate yourself. If you can't find everything you need in this book, there are many others that offer sympathetic perspectives on kinky sex. The Internet too is a prime source for information, advice, and support on virtually every aspect of kinky sex. The more you learn, the safer you will feel and the greater your self-confidence will grow.

Another good way to get comfortable is to talk to your partner in as much depth as you can about what he or she likes, why he or she likes it, where he or she thinks the desire comes from, and so on. Encourage your partner to share childhood memories (Did your partner enjoy playing "pirate" or other capture and bondage games as a kid? Did he or she ever dress up in fetishistic garments or shoes?). Share fantasies and discuss possible scenarios you might be willing to enact. Don't be afraid to ask a lot of "what ifs?" and "how comes?"

If your partner is asking you to try something new, then he or she must be willing to spend time discussing it with you in depth. Make this a team effort. Your partner can work with you, guiding you and giving you as much time, information, and support as you need.

If you're worried that your partner will expect you to take the kink to a point that frightens you, discuss using a "safe word" (you will find a full definition of this term in the glossary on page 318): This allows you to stop the kinky play when you've reached your limit. Even if you are the dominant in the power equation, you have a right to stop when it gets too intense for you.

A fun way to learn to relax is with trial runs. Let's say your partner has a fantasy about wearing nipple clips. Long before you attach those clips, visit an adult toy store together and look at various kinds. Have store clerks explain how they work. Clerks in these stores are occupationally blasé and talk about bizarre sex aids as casually as a cheese merchant explains the difference between Gouda and Brie. Feel free to ask as many questions as you like. Someone who sells nipple clips is not about to judge someone who may buy them.

Don't put yourself under pressure to buy something on this first trip. Let the idea sink in for a while before you spend your money. You can always return another time.

If you'd really like to be silly, you can even buy a pair of clips and attach them to a stuffed animal when you get home. After seeing a pair of nipple clips on your teddy bear for a week or so, trust me, they become a lot less intimidating.

Finally, try to see the fetish or kink with new eyes. Using the nipple clips example again, think about what purpose they really serve. In effect, nipple clips are a convenient device to pinch and stimulate your lover's nipples so your hands are free to move on to other things. That doesn't sound so bad, does it?

Kinky sex is what you make it. Treat it like a shameful, guilty vice that must remain hidden and you will never see the joy in it. Make it a playful adventure into expanding your erotic horizons as a team and you'll find that it can bring you closer together, not just sexually but emotionally.

## 2. Focus on Your Partner

Do you care deeply about your partner? Do you want him or her to have the absolute best sex with you and you alone? Does it turn you on to see your partner excited?

For most people, male and female alike, knowing that our partners are incredibly turned on by the things we do to them, with them, and for them in bed is a turn-on in itself.

If you answered "yes" to the three questions above, then you will find it very satisfying to watch your partner's reactions when you act out one of his or her kinky fantasies.

One mistake people make is when they focus uniquely on the fantasy activity, almost forgetting, in the moment, that they are sharing an intimate experience with the one they love. Because they don't quite understand the fetish or kink, and because the things we don't understand seem threatening, they may create an emotional wall between themselves and the unknown.

This kind of distancing is negative and hurtful: Your partner will sense that you are uninterested without knowing why. And you are creating a negative feedback loop for yourself that may ultimately make you unwilling to fulfill your partner's needs.

For example, let's say for the heck of it that your partner has been asking you to wear latex to bed. If you take a passive approach and wear the latex, hoping that it will be over quickly so you can get on to the good stuff, you will miss out entirely on the complete experience.

Instead of thinking about how nice it was of you to wear the latex, or how hot it's getting inside the latex, or any of the other weird thoughts people have when they distance themselves from what they are doing, focus on how your partner is responding to you. Look for the familiar signs of excitement that turn you on when you're having more conventional sex. The faint smell of sweat, the flush of sexual heat radiating from your lover's skin, the happy sighs and groans, the hardness or wetness of your partner—let yourself enjoy those familiar, intimate aspects of your sex life together. Those responses will also let you know that you are the most exciting person in your partner's life.

## 3. Focus on Yourself

Now that you've seen the effect the kinky act has had on your partner, look into yourself for connections.

A good place to start is by trying to identify what it is that you, personally, really love about sex with your partner. Do you enjoy slow sensuality? Are you intrigued by the roles people play, or the way one partner surrenders to the other? Perhaps your turn-on comes from the raw sensuality of naked bodies rubbing together.

This time, I'll use bondage as an example. Your partner requested that you put her in tight rope bondage. You've done it all safely (because you've read chapter 5 in this book on bondage, right?), you've paid careful attention to all her reactions, and you are (one hopes) pleased to see that she is panting in wild excitement.

So what's in it for you, now that you've tied all the ropes?

For starters, you can revert to familiar fun, such as foreplay, with manual or oral stimulation of her breasts and genitals. If the person tied up is male, and the only part of him still moving is his erection . . . well, need I tell you what to do next? If you like oral sex, your bound partner probably will soon be liking it too.

Or perhaps there is some little spot you've never had a chance to explore before. Now's your big chance.

The point here is that in kinky sex, as in life, 50/50 is only fair. Once you've given your partner his or her fantasy scenario, you have earned the right to be a litte selfish. Use this is an opportunity to express your passion for your partner in ways that give you the greatest physical pleasure.

## 4. Make the Emotional Connection

The fourth step is the hardest, but the most logical one. The physical side of things is important, but so is the emotional side. You need to make the emotional connection between what your partner gets out of a kinky experience and the kinds of things that turn you on.

You will find that, whether we're kinky or vanilla, we all want the same basic things from sex. We want to feel loved, stimulated, desired, and we want to love, stimulate, and desire. While conventional sex may provide all those things for you, your partner may need a special sensation or a particular scenario to feel those same things.

One of the most rewarding aspects of enacting your lover's sexual fantasies is seeing how happy and excited your partner becomes. If you know your partners' deepest sexual secrets and needs, you essentially possess the key to unlocking their sexual passions. All of us have moments of insecurity in bed: We may fear that our partner doesn't find us attractive anymore or that our skills or sexual performance is inadequate. It is truly an incredible emotional rush to know you hold the key to sexually satisfying your partner as no one else ever has.

## KINK AND GOD: THE SPIRITUAL CONFLICT

*I've been reading about D&S on the Internet. I know this is what is missing from my life. Do you have any ideas on how I can get my husband to dominate me? I told him I wanted to be his submissive but he is very religious (we are Christians) and said it was a sin. What am I going to do? I need this.*

Whatever our religious training, most of us were taught, from an early age, strict rules about what we may and may not do in bed. If your husband has tried to be true to such rules all his life, he may not be ready or willing to change. Indeed, to him such change could represent a flight from his faith.

Religions on the whole (and particularly in their most orthodox expressions) view sex as a reproductive duty, not as something one does for fun. So any kind of sex for pleasure is usually treated as "dirty" and less legitimate an expression of adult sexuality than missionary-position intercourse.

Many believers abide by the strictures set by their faith, no matter how tough those limits are. The support they get from family, fellow worshippers, and clergy constantly reinforces their ideas about sex and reassures them that they've made the best moral choice. Whether you agree with them or not, their beliefs should be respected. After all, if you can't respect their beliefs, you can't expect them to respect yours.

You will also find some believers who feel that any and all views that differ from theirs are evil; in some cases, they may perceive a partner's request to try something different as an attempt to lead them into sin. Such people cannot and will not violate their spiritual beliefs for the sake of physical gratification—neither yours nor their own.

However, it is also undeniable that more and more people are finding it difficult to live up to standards set by rabbis, priests, ministers, and imams. We may seek out religions that are more accepting of sexual diversity; we may, sadly, lead secret lives, torn between what we secretly crave and what our faith demands; or we may turn away from religion entirely.

The rift between the standards held up by religions and our natural sexual impulses creates emotional conflicts that undermine our self-esteem, spoil our relationships, and even hurt our performance in bed. It's difficult to have fun in bed when you're afraid you'll go to hell for it.

A few years ago, I was counseling someone who'd undergone surgery for prostate cancer. Predictably, he was having problems with impotence, a not uncommon result of the surgery. His urologist had prescribed a rather clumsy device to help him maintain an erection. My client complained that by the time he managed to get the contraption on, his wife had either dozed off or lost all interest.

I recommended that, to help ease the postsurgical transition, they vary their sexual routine and emphasize other forms of sex-play, such as mutual masturbation and oral sex. He told me that since he and his wife were fundamentalist Christians, this went against everything they had been taught. He did not feel comfortable raising the subject with her and was sure she would be mortified if he did. He preferred to do without sex (despite having had a very active, happy sex life with his wife until his surgery) rather than try something other than intercourse.

With such prohibitions against sex acts that many active adults consider well within the norm of intimate relations, you can imagine the conflicts that SM and fetishism create for believers. Still, many can and do make peace with their kinky needs. Some view sexual differences not as a curse but a gift from God that enables them to enjoy a wide range of sensation. Others note that the Bible does not specifically condemn unusual sex acts within a monogamous relationship. (Indeed, the Song of Solomon contains more than a few kinky verses.) And some folks simply take the humanistic attitude that anything that occurs in private is acceptable within the context of a loving, devoted relationship.

Times are changing and so are the attitudes of some clergypeople. Not long ago, I was invited to speak to an SM/fetish discussion club. To my surprised delight, a group of about eight ministers suddenly filed in and occupied a front row. They were young, progressive, and evidently open to outreach from the SM community. They had come to hear what I had to say in hopes of learning something that would help them minister to the kinky members of their flocks.

Among the many fascinating developments on the Internet is the recent emergence of Web sites devoted to reconciling Christian faith with kinky sex. I recently visited one, simply titled "Christian BDSM," which provides a scholarly framework to defend and explain how heterosexual male domination is not at odds with the teachings of Jesus Christ but rather in accordance with certain basic Christian beliefs. (Most notably, that men be a "cover" to women.) Meanwhile, on these sites' message boards, you will also find discussions by submissive males, males with gay fantasies, and so on, all of whom are seeking answers through their faith to the sexual orientation they recognize within themselves.

Whatever your religious convictions, the most important task ahead is to try to open communications between yourself and your partner, in hopes that you can reach a compromise you will both find morally acceptable. To help you get started, I've prepared a list of five key talking points.

## Talking Points on Sex and God

1. *Talk about your own struggles.* It is helpful for your partner to know that you have sought answers, and important for your partner to understand the seriousness and depth of your needs. A person's sexual identity is generally formed by the time she or he is five years old. Whether or not we ever find peace with it, our sexual persona will be with us until the end of our lives. If you can learn to accept yourself as you are, you will be better able to teach your partner to accept you as well.

Let your partner know that in order to really love you—the whole you, the intimate, honest you, and not just that side of you that you let the world see—he or she must begin to accept that your kinky desires are as much a part of your personality as your sense of humor, your moods, and so on.

2. *Talk about a compassionate God.* If you are both believers, stress that your sexual needs are another aspect of the complete person that God created. This approach can be very comforting as it embraces the notion of a supreme being who creates people in a spirit of love and understanding and who wants people to derive happiness from the lives they were given. The variations in sexual needs may then be viewed as part of a supreme being's plan for your life. Since we do not yet know just how sexual identity is formed, "God made me this way" is as good an explanation as any. Of course, this doesn't remove from your shoulders the responsibility for leading a moral life, but it does emphasize that a person can be moral and kinky at the same time.

Your strongest suit here is quite simply that, despite the difficulty of having this conversation, you are so committed to your relationship that you are willing to open yourself up to possible criticism.

It's also good to point out that while your confession of kinkiness may be new, your interest in kink is not. In effect, the person your partner has been living with all along was always kinky, just reluctant or afraid to say so. You are still the same wonderful person your partner fell in love with; you are just trying, now, to open your heart completely and to find a new, higher level of happiness in your relationship.

3. *Stress your commitment to your partner.* People often make the mistake of putting the emphasis on their sexual needs without putting it in the context of their relationship. They say things like "I want to do this" instead of "I want to do this with you." If you love your partner, let him or her know that any variations you add to your sex life are an extension of that love.

It's to be expected that some partners will feel deeply threatened when you tell them about your sexual fantasies. They may feel betrayed that you've kept them a secret for so long; or they may, for a time, feel that you aren't the person they thought they married. This is, by no means, an easy phase for a couple, but it is, for better or worse, a typical one. Couples can get past it with time and patience.

Emphasize that you are turning to your partner for comfort, support, and understanding because you *are* still in love and because you *do* want your relationship to continue, hopefully on even happier terms. Make your partner feel as included and desired as you can. Whether your partner is male or female, reassurance that the fundamentals of your relationship haven't changed will help keep him or her from thinking you've changed.

4. *Find a spiritual context for your needs.* If you are submissive, explore the spiritual aspects of your needs. The need to worship, obey, and serve a higher authority should strike a resonant chord in a religious partner of any faith. Try to frame your sexual needs within the context of a devoted relationship, where

The Kink in All of Us 65

serving your partner's needs is part of your spiritual aspirations. Without being blasphemous, you may be able to explain that you see your partner as closer than you to God, and that by serving him (or her), you are serving God—something most submissives find to be true. Love of a dominant does not replace love of God, but certainly can be seen as an adjunct to it.

Female submissives dealing with religious men (and vice versa) already have a religious context for the man being the one in charge, sexually and otherwise.

If you are dominant, you will need to determine on your own whether and if there is an existing religious framework for your sexual needs. Again, most religions support the concept of male dominance. Female dominants, however—unless they and their partners are pagan or believe in a female supreme being—will have to give this issue deeper thought. However, most Judeo-Christian sects do recognize women as decision-makers and leaders in the home. If you already take charge of many of the important household decisions; if you run the kitchen, the children, and the general life of the family, you may be able to talk about naturally extending your leadership role into the bedroom.

5. *Practice forgiveness.* This is a two-way street. Try to forgive your partner if he or she at first reacts with shock or criticism. Give your partner room to fail, and also the forgiveness to redeem him- or herself. In other words, try to give your partner everything that you are hoping to get, and more.

If your partner has been completely faithful to his or her religious ideals since childhood, it will take time for a change to occur. Don't expect an overnight epiphany. You are going to be dealing with a lifetime of lessons, inhibitions, and fears about the dangers of going against the grain. It's possible your partner will need to go through a slow spiritual evolution to overcome his or her prejudices before being able to fully comprehend that what you are asking for is acceptable.

The best thing you can do is to help educate your partner and to encourage him or her to see this as a growth experience for you both, spiritually and otherwise. Use kink-positive books as tools for communication. If your spiritual leader—priest, rabbi, minister, or other cleric—is sympathetic or at least non-judgmental, ask for counseling. If you are on the Internet, seek out others who, like you, are believers who have successfully incorporated kink into their lives. Look for positive role models wherever you can.

Meanwhile, keep your own spirits up by reminding yourself that if you can ultimately get what you need from the one you love, the wait is worthwhile. The most meaningful satisfaction for you, though, should be the knowledge that by doing this you are attempting to live in truth. No spiritual endeavor is higher than that.

## CHAPTER FOUR

# *Getting Involved*

## KINK AND THE SINGLE PERVERT

*I just reentered the single world after a fourteen-year marriage to a totally vanilla woman. Now that I'm free again, I have decided I have to pursue my lifelong dream of being a sex slave. From what I see on the Internet, I know there is a whole big world out there of people like me. Can you tell me where to find a dominatrix or give me the name of one of your dominant girlfriends?*

Over the years, I've received hundreds of letters from men and women begging me to match them up with submissives or dominants. The Jewish mother part of me would honestly like to start a second career as a sadomasochistic matchmaker. Fortunately, that is only a very small part of me.

Instead, I give everyone the same answer. I tell them to connect with any of the hundreds of membership organizations, educational outreach groups, Internet message boards, and Web sites all geared to the social needs of kinky people.

I won't lie: Being kinky and single can be tough on the ego. As hard as it is for vanilla people to find suitable mates, finding Mr. or Ms. Right Pervert is even harder. First, kinky singles have a smaller pool of potential partners to draw from. There are fewer kinky people than there are straight people. Beyond that, kinky sex rouses so many different (and often negative) responses, that a lot of eligible kinksters would rather not date at all than risk rejection or waste their time on people who cannot comprehend their needs.

The good news, though, is that a huge social structure exists within the kink communities. You may not meet your ideal mate at an SM club or in a BDSM chat-group on the Net, but you will be able to make contacts with nice, friendly people. Sometimes it's just comforting to know that there are other normal people out there who enjoy the same kinks as you do.

Still, the kinky subculture isn't for everyone. Thousands of the people who've contacted me identify themselves as middle-class, mainstream individuals—businesspeople, college professors, lawyers, programmers, office workers. They aren't prepared to visit SM clubs. They don't want their names on SM mailing lists. They just want to find a kinky person to love.

There is nothing wrong with this.

The Scene has its purposes. For one, it provides social opportunities for kinky people through its numerous organizations and clubs. But it is not the be-all and end-all of kinky sex. In other words, you don't have to join the Scene to find the kinky lover of your dreams. The fact is that wherever you go, no matter how small or remote your community, there are other kinky people in your area. This is a simple statistical reality. The challenge is connecting with them.

Frankly, the kinky subculture would just as soon not have everyone with a kinky fantasy rushing to join their ranks. The phenomenal growth of the SM/fetish Scene in the past ten years has placed enormous stress on resources. Many of the old-timers now worry that novices might be hurt because the Scene just can't meet the demands of all the newcomers who need to be educated on how to do SM safely and on the ethical rules that serious players live by. (For a summary of those, jump ahead to the final chapter and look under "Ten Rules to Remember," page 285.)

In this section of the book, I cover basic ground rules for getting involved, both for those who want to explore the SM/fetish Scene and those who don't. (Don't forget to flip to the glossary in the appendix for definitions of kinky terms you don't understand.)


## GETTING KINKY

*I've been dating a man for six weeks and it's reaching that point where I feel I need to decide whether or not to tell him my fan-*

*tasies about whipping and tight bondage. So why aren't I doing it? To be honest, I'm scared. I don't want to frighten him away but at the same time I know that if he can't deal with them, there's no point getting more involved with him. Maybe part of me is afraid of finding out that we're doomed. My biggest worry, I guess, is rejection. When I told my ex-boyfriend what turned me on, he freaked out. That's why he is "ex." What should I do?*

I am a great believer in direct speech and direct action, but even I would hesitate to launch into a full description of my most cherished kinky fantasies with someone until I felt reasonably certain that he was kinky too. I don't see the point in revealing such private thoughts to someone with whom I won't be sexually intimate. And if he isn't kinky, we won't be sexually intimate.

Just as people are entitled to be kinky, they are also entitled not to be kinky. It's hard to remember that after one has gone out on an emotional limb by confessing precious sexual secrets. If you feel anxious or guilty about your desires, it's only natural that you would feel angry, frustrated, or ashamed when someone turns you down, even though you may know in your head that the other person has a right to choose a different sexual path for himself.

Instead of taking the direct approach, I recommend that you try the following low-key techniques to check on a potential partner's "kinkability."

## YE OLDE SUBTLE HINTES

### Kinky Flirting

A submissive man I know once told me the story of how he met his mistress. He was at an expensive bar in an upscale part of town, waiting for friends to arrive. A good-looking woman in a business suit sat next to him and they chatted casually. Before long, he offered to buy her a drink. She accepted and jokingly commented about how eager he seemed to please. He joked back, "I live to serve." She looked him in the eye, then told him that if he meant it, he should get down on his knees then and there and kiss her feet. He did.

And they lived happily ever after.

There are lots of little ways—most of them a lot tamer than what my friends did—to let someone know that you swing a certain way. Can you squeeze in a little reference to something naughty? Can you find a moment when a lighthearted joke about kink would be appropriate? Grasping someone's elbow and breathing "I want to be your slave!" doesn't count. On the other hand, if you're submissive, acting sweet and eager to please might get the message across.

Just don't try so hard to let someone know where you're coming from that they leave. This applies to dominants too. You can scare away people who might actually be aroused by kink but who are not prepared to talk about it just yet. Give it time, drop your hints, and see if anything takes. If your friend is still giving you blank looks (or, worse, hostile ones) after several dates, you need to face the fact that this person is not going to be your ideal kinky mate.

## Body Language

Yes, body language rears its head once again. Most people can lie with their words; far fewer can lie with their bodies. So, without gawking, watch the way your friend responds to your kinky flirtations. Is she clenching her fists? Have veins popped out in his head from all the jaw-clenching he's doing? These are not good signs. On the other hand, if your companion seems relaxed, amused, or aroused, or if he or she leans forward or (better still) touches you, those are excellent signs.

If you see them, *keep flirting!* When and if you become physically intimate, it will be natural to begin putting some of those naughty ideas you shared into practice.

## Books

Perhaps the safest and least provocative way to see whether a partner may be interested in kinky sex is by introducing them to books about kinky sex. Do feel free to share this book, of course. But if there are any classics you love, I suppose that would be acceptable too. If you don't know of any, never fear: Chapter 13 contains a list of popular titles. Books can open the way to fruitful and revealing conversations.

Please don't thrust a book into each new partner's hand and ask for a book report. That makes reading an obligation for them instead of the shared pleasure it should be. Aim for a little finesse.

A submissive woman I know always initiates conversations about books with prospective boyfriends. Beginning with tame titles, she eventually works her way up to her favorite SM book, *Story of O*. If her partner has read the book, she finds out very quickly how he felt about it. If he hated it, she stops the conversation there. If he loved it, she knows she's found a kindred spirit. And if he hasn't read it, but seems intrigued, she will lend him a copy.

This approach protects her dignity. She never needs to get graphic about what she wants but you would have to be brain-dead not to see where she's going. Plus, it is emotionally safer to have someone reject a book rather than oneself.

You can use movies, television shows, or any other pop-culture references in the same way. For example, a lot of people were turned on by the old TV series *The Avengers* because of the fetish clothes and frequent bondage scenarios. If you'd like ideas on books or movies you can mention, chapter 13 contains a ton of references to get you started.

## Kinky Chemistry

This isn't exactly a hint (or even a "hinte"). It is an observation I've made about myself over decades of shameless cavorting. Almost invariably, any man for whom I've felt intense sexual passion has turned out to be kinky. We may not have done explicitly kinky things or ever discussed kink openly. But, in retrospect, the men who really made my toes curl were always sexually weird.

Obviously, this is not a scientific method of judging a partner's kink-potential.

You must be very careful not to convince yourself that someone is kinky just because you want him to be, or to believe that because you are attracted to him, he must therefore be attracted to you. Don't think that because you're kinky and he's kinky you're destined to live happily ever after in unadulterated bliss, either.

However, if you are kinky and if your partner gets to you in a way that few other people ever have, and if you seem to inspire a similar fever of lust in this person, I'd say it's an encouraging sign that you have complementary sexual desires. Indeed, this is what true sexual chemistry is all about.

## A WORD ABOUT TIMING

If you know you need kink to feel sexually complete, if you are an adult, and if you seek a long-term or permanent relationship, then there is no reason to wait for months before raising the topic of kink with a potential mate.

Sexual compatibility is key to every joyous union. Just as you'd look for someone who shares your feelings and values about family, children, religion, and so on, you should try to find out, right up front, if you share the same sexual values. Do this before either of you makes commitments, and definitely before you fall in love.

This does not mean you must act on your desires right away. It only means that you need to share those books and movies sooner rather than later.

If you do not intend to have sex until you marry, at least try to discuss your future intimacy with your fiancé, so that you don't find out on your wedding night that you married someone who believes you'll burn in hell for wearing see-through panties.

If you wait until you've forged strong emotional bonds or signed a marriage license, it will seem shallow and selfish to dump people who won't indulge a fetish you didn't tell them about in the first place.

It will seem that way because it is.

Your happiness is your responsibility. It is also your moral responsibility not to make someone else miserable as you pursue your happiness. Limit the potential emotional damage to yourself and people you care about by clarifying these issues before you promise to stick by them forever.

## PLAYING IT SAFE AND KEEPING IT CONSENSUAL

Here are four essential thinking points for everyone who is beginning an SM relationship.

### 1. Who Is This Person I Am About to Play With?

This is the simplest and most basic question to ask in any relationship, yet it is one many newcomers to BDSM never even consider. Many people assume that if they are attending a well-known club, or a party organized by a reputable group, all the people they will meet are trustworthy. This is neither a safe nor a healthy assumption.

The greatest disasters inevitably occur when the people involved don't have a clear knowledge of who the other person is, what that person's history has been in the world of SM, and whether that person is, in all respects, a trustworthy, decent human being. The sad reality is that, as interest in BDSM expands, more and more people who are positively clueless about conducting their SM relationships in a safe and consensual fashion join clubs and attend parties.

Never forget that SM and abuse are no more related than intercourse and rape. The only difference between a dominant who forces others to do things that upset and terrify them and a criminal is that no one has called the police on that dominant . . . yet. Responsible people in the SM Scene deplore all instances of nonconsensual force and report crimes of violence to the police.

### 2. How Do I Know Whom to Trust?

There is simply no substitute for the tried-and-true method one would use for all romantic relationships: You must take the time to get to know the person. If you think you know someone well enough to put your full trust in him or her after a few dates or some sexy E-mails, you are kidding yourself.

If you're looking for a long-term or permanent relationship, I recommend what I like to call "D&S dating." As in regular dating, you spend time doing real-world things together— going to movies, having dinner together, visiting museums, or any other normal, social activity as a couple. The difference between D&S dating and regular dating is that instead of making out or making love at evening's end, you do kinky things together. (Of course, you can still make out and make love too!)

Dating for a couple of months gives you and your potential partner the opportunity to see one another in a wide variety of circumstances. If, in the course of dating, you discover that, for example, he or she tends to lie or fudge the truth about things; that he is irresponsible and thoughtless; that she plays games or blows hot and cold; or any other traits that turn you off, then the dating ends, and you are not locked into any commitments.

It may seem slow, but the rewards are that by the time you are ready to make a commitment you really know the person. You know how they react to situations, you know the way their mind works, and, ideally, you have grown quite fond of them.

### 3. That's So Complicated! Can't I Ever Play with Strangers?

Of course you can, if you take the right precautions. In fact, that's what safe words were created for: to limit the risk of unintentional harm when doing SM with casual partners.

The real question is not whether you can or cannot play with strangers; it is whether you are able to make a sane choice for yourself about how much trust you will give up to someone you don't know very well. You must be very careful not to give trust up too freely, particularly if you are the romantic, impulsive type who is likely to become smitten overnight and liable to say almost anything when aroused.

For some people, the urge to do SM is overwhelming, particularly if their feelings have been bottled up for a long time. But the plain fact is that there are no shortcuts in SM. If you want a quality relationship, you must invest the time and make a commitment to yourself not to settle for or to jump at every opportunity that comes along. Not all opportunities are equal. Some can lead to significant emotional pain. Others are downright dangerous.

To protect yourself, limit your risk. Don't give carte blanche consent to people you haven't known for a significant amount of time (a basic rule of thumb might be three months). Meanwhile, though the network isn't as reliable as it once was, if you met this person at an SM party, club, group meeting, or any other SM venue (including online environments), you should be able to find at least one and possibly more people who know this person. Ask them for feedback.

There is nothing rude or disrespectful about asking people whether they know another player or have ever seen them in action. If the person you want to play with expresses anger, fear, resentment, or any other negative emotions about your talking to others, then that's a warning that something is not right.

People who are comfortable with themselves and proud of their reputations for safe, consensual behavior will not be offended by you checking on their background. Sane and caring individuals expect new partners to be cautious.

Finally, if you are considering visiting a professional dominant, chapter 11 offers a complete discussion on how to decide which ones are safe, and what you can expect when you go.

### 4. But Won't My Safe Word Protect Me?

Not necessarily.

The most endearing characteristics of sexual submissives— particularly their eagerness to please—are precisely what abusers prey on. I've heard horror stories about submissives whose dominants threatened never to see them again if they used their safe word, or who otherwise bullied submissives into accepting much harsher treatment than they wanted. If your casual partner turns out to be an idiot or a creep, he or she may not even stop when you use your safe word.

Safe words are designed to protect dominants as well, yet they too must be cautious. Not all submissives are trustworthy or genuine. Some subs will use safe words to control or manipulate a scene, rather than to indicate when they've reached a genuine limit. One of the most troubling situations is when a submissive refrains from using a safe word when he or she should. This leads the dominant to believe that everything is fine, only to discover hours, days, or months later that the submissive feels the dominant went too far.

Why would a sub not use a safe word? Sometimes it's naïveté or the desire to please. Other times it's stubborn pride. Some masochists set out to prove to themselves that they can take anything a dominant dishes out, and it becomes an ego trip for them to tolerate suffering. Still others are so hungry to live out their fantasies that they would rather put up with a bad relationship than be alone. Whatever their reasons, bottom/submissive partners who don't use their safe words when they should are courting disaster.

Bottom line: Whether you are top or bottom, dominant or submissive, never let a safe word lull you into a false sense of security. It is a tool for safer play, not a guarantee of it.

## WHERE TO GO, WHO TO DO

If you feel you'd like to explore the SM Scene, this section will familiarize you with the social network of organizations and events that draw together kinky people.

All the major U.S. cities (and dozens of smaller ones) have at least one kinky club. These groups typically hold meetings where people talk about kinky sex in a low-pressure environment. Hundreds of regional, national, and international SM/fetish events also occur annually throughout the world. Most of these venues welcome newcomers and will help orient you safely to the world of kinky sex.

### Making Contacts

The Internet is the best source for kinky information, advice, and adult entertainment. There are sites where kinky people can place free personal ads, chat-groups and kinky IRC channels, pages hosted by BDSM/fetish groups throughout the world, and an endless variety of private and commercial sites devoted to exploring the mysteries and explaining the methods of doing kink. I have a comprehensive Internet resource guide to kink on my site (gloria-brame.com). This guide will steer you to thousands of hand-selected kinky venues.

The Net has proven invaluable to people who don't live in major cities, or who cannot otherwise go to SM clubs or events. While there is no absolute guarantee of anonymity, you are certainly better able to protect your identity online than off. Meanwhile, you broaden the pool of potential kinky partners online because you can hook up with people around the world. This can create problems if you find someone who lives thousands of miles away from you, but love has a way of solving those problems. Hundreds, if not thousands, of couples have met online and relocated for the sake of true kinky love.

If you don't have access to the Net, then you will have to find people the old-fashioned way: by turning to magazines and newspapers. In major cities, check out a large, liberal newsstand, a gay/lesbian bookstore, or adult sex shops that stock periodicals. Look for kinky magazines that have real editorial content—not the porn mags that contain nothing but erotic fiction and pictures. *Skin Two, Ritual, Secret, Marquis, The Leather Journal, Drummer,* and *SandMutopian Guardian* are among the numerous kink-oriented journals that appeal to literate readers, and they all contain articles and ads about the organized Scene.

Big-city alternative papers (like *New York Express,* Boston's *Phoenix,* Atlanta's *Creative Loafing,* Washington, D.C.'s *City Paper,* and so on) accept kinky personals and sometimes ads for SM services. Another possibility are "adult entertainment" rags. You won't be reading them for editorial content, but they do often list kinky clubs and events.

## Six Types of Kinky Venues

Although the kinky subculture is a complex, mysterious world, filled with its own traditions, rituals, customs, rules, and slang, it can also be a very warm and welcoming place for novices. Some groups, such as the Til Eulenspiegel Society (TES) in New York

City, make a point of reaching out to newcomers, and run special educational programs to meet their needs.

Here is a primer on social organizations and kinky venues you could attend.

1. *Kinky Education/Support Membership Groups:* The basic purpose of most membership groups is to provide a friendly, structured environment in which people can get support for their issues, talk about the diversity of kinky sexuality, and make friends.

Each SM organization has something slightly different to offer. Some, like the network of "PEP" (People Exchanging Power) clubs, welcome the paying public to weekly meetings that combine lectures and safety demonstrations with parties. The Til Eulenspiegel Society (TES) in New York offers different programs for focus groups (newcomers, people of color, male dominant/female submissive couples, and so on). Other groups focus uniquely on education and host parties or bar nights only on special occasions. Or they may sponsor free educational outreach programs for the public but restrict parties to members only. And so on.

New members are usually allowed to attend meetings for a nominal fee. The only requirement is that you be sincerely interested in learning about kink. Unless the event has been advertised as a party, everyone will likely be wearing street clothes and the environment will be fairly relaxed. There is almost always a leader, or a few leaders, who will make announcements and moderate the program.

There will be an opportunity, after the formal part of the evening ends, for you to mingle with others, although no one is required to do so. Some groups will ask people to sit in a circle and to talk briefly about why they came to the meeting. You are not required to participate if it makes you uneasy. If you do, and they ask for your name, it is acceptable to use a pseudonym (also known as a "Scene name").

Do not go to one of these meetings expecting to find sex. These meetings can be surprisingly respectable, and polite behavior is required of all who attend. This means: no ogling, no lewd remarks, no aggressive come-ons, no sleazy propositions.

Strange but true, an SM/fetish group is a far more civilized place than a singles' bar.

2. *SM Bars and Clubs:* Most major American cities, coast to coast, have at least one or two clubs that cater to the local SM/leather population. In smaller cities, the only places that may cater to kinky people are likely to be gay establishments. Some of them restrict entry to gays and bisexuals. However, more and more traditionally gay-only SM clubs have been opening their doors to all SM/fetish people, regardless of orientation.

If you go to a bar, you may see a lot of people in leather and denim. They will mostly be standing around, drinking beer and chatting, dancing, or playing pinball. Unless it's a party night, chances are you won't see anything wilder than that. The atmosphere does, however, change considerably on party nights and on weekends, when such bars are packed. Then it's possible that somewhere in a back room (or even under a table) someone may be doing highly naughty things with someone else.

An SM club, unlike a bar, is, by definition, wild. You will see large-scale equipment (racks, cages, crosses, etc.), and you will see people using them. Because of safe-sex concerns, you probably won't see sex acts, but you may see nudity, bare-bottomed spankings, whippings, foot worship, and other things. You are under no obligation whatsoever to participate, but be aware that just about anything could be going on at your elbow at any given moment. If you are put off by the sight of people publicly engaged in kinky acts, then don't go. This is part of the culture of public play-spaces and the reason why many people attend them.

People don't go to SM clubs to drink beer because most SM clubs do not serve alcohol. Partly this is because most Scene people feel that SM and alcohol do not mix, and partly it's because, in most states, nudity is not allowed where alcohol is served. Visitors come to these clubs to meet people, to act out fantasies, or to watch SM in action. So if you go, be prepared both for soft drinks and sights you won't forget.

3. *Fund-Raisers:* SM organizations frequently run events to raise money for important SM community causes. Sometimes it's just a beer night at a bar. But often there will be some special feature to entertain or amuse the crowd. It might be an SM writer reading from a book, or it could be "booths" where you can buy tickets for the booth operator to give you anything from a back rub to a spanking. I recently attended a fund-raiser where a young man was bound securely to a table and whipped to arousal. Then his erection was used for ring toss.

If that isn't amusing, I don't know what is.

Fund-raisers charge an entrance fee; you may also be asked to contribute money or to participate in an auction of merchandise. Fund-raisers are a great opportunity to talk to and observe kinky people while helping to support a good cause.

4. *Leatherfests and Fetish Fairs:* Throughout the year, various organizations host the SM equivalent of a business convention—but with a few kinky twists. These events typically feature a full weekend of activities: panels and workshops led by Scene activists and teachers, SM demonstrations, a vendor fair, a charitable auction, parties, and leather contests. These events draw anywhere from fifty to several thousand people, depending on location and the prestige of the sponsoring organizations.

You can also find "fetish fairs" in a few major cities. Imagine an open-air flea market devoted to kinky merchandise and you've got the general idea. They're an excellent way to safely mingle in a public space. They're also free of charge. The largest and best known of these is the Folsom Street Fair, which is held each fall in San Francisco. In 1998, over a quarter of a million people attended that SM block party. Boston and New York have begun offering similar events, though on a smaller scale.

Leather contests are another type of get-together for the kinky generation. However, social opportunities are limited during the contest itself because the emphasis is on the people onstage. There will be some mingling in the lobby, before the program begins, but that's about it.

Contests take place in a theater setting. Contestants are judged in several areas, including their knowledge of

SM/leather history, their ability to script and choreograph a theatrical SM "demo," and their ability to articulate the philosophy of safe, consensual kinky sex.

While some of these competitions were once gay- or lesbian-only, you can now expect to find people of all orientations attending and competing. Be prepared for diversity.

Some of the more prestigious competitions are International Mr./Ms. Leather (IML and IMsL), Mr. Drummer (sponsored by the gay magazine of the same name), and International Master/Slave. There are regional preliminary contests for all of the above; the winners move on to the national or international level.

At these contests, people compete for the opportunity to be officially endorsed representatives of the SM/leather communities. Winners travel around the country, lecture to groups, appear at fund-raisers, and do good works in support of educating the public about safe, sane, consensual SM.

5. *Play Parties:* These range from small, intimate gatherings where an individual may invite friends to his or her home, to large-scale parties sponsored by clubs or membership organizations. The purpose of a play party is to give kinky people a chance to live out some of their fantasies in the presence of others.

Since these are largely by-invitation-only events, you will need to know someone to get in. Your best bet is to join a group that hosts play parties or to make friends with people who attend them.

If you should snag an invitation, try to find out in advance what will be going on. Will there be nudity? Will you be expected to participate? Although no one is required to participate at a play party, it is assumed that you came there because you were open to the idea of joining in. It's quite possible you may end up spending the entire evening just watching others, but it's equally possible that someone may approach you and propose that you play together.

If this possibility alarms you but you still feel you want to explore this option, ask the person who invited you if he or she will be your mentor for the night and handle any sticky situations, should they arise. Asking "Will you protect me?" works fine too. If the person turns you down, then you need some new friends.

6. *Advanced Perversion:* You've joined a group, you've attended a leather event, you've been to an SM club. What else is new under the sun?

If you live in a big city, you may be able to find a club that occasionally hosts "slave auctions." This playful kinky group game has always been popular in the New York SM Scene, where the infamous Hellfire Club regularly runs them for the entertainment of patrons.

Slave auctions work more or less as follows.

Throughout the early part of the evening, the DJ will periodically announce that a slave auction will take place at a specified hour (usually late). Sometimes they limit contestants to submissives or bottoms only, but just as often they will allow dominants to get up and auction off a "scene."

There will be a roster for you to sign; on it, you specify what kind of fetishes or kinks you are offering. You are not expected to get into all the details of your fantasies, but instead to give potential bidders a few ideas about what you would like, whether it's foot worship, bondage, spankings, or anything else.

When the auction begins, the DJ will call people up one by one to a stage. I've seen newbies freeze like deer in headlights, but uninhibited types really enjoy this opportunity to present themselves as a hot commodity. Subs may strip off their clothes (particularly if friends from the audience urge them on); doms may roll their whips and glare menacingly. It is up to each contestant to decide how much or little they want to do.

It's hard to predict just who will create a bidding war but, generally speaking, unattached female submissives create something of a frenzy. What a surprise.

I recall, though, attending one auction at Hellfire where a handsome young man, and a complete newcomer to the Scene, listed in his description that he was *really* embarrassed at the thought of having to take off his clothes in public. The dominatrices in attendance went hog-wild over that gent.

The audience bids with play money—little colored coupons the club prints up. Sometimes you can pay cash for coupons but more often you "earn" the play money each time you buy a soft drink at the bar. Occasionally, people will just hand you money for no reason except mischievousness. When I was first starting out, I was quite surprised and touched that a submissive man kept stuffing coupons into my hands. His nefarious plot was revealed when the auction began: He wanted me to win him, the scamp.

Another way of earning play money is by entering the auction yourself—you get to keep whatever people paid for you. My would-be slave had apparently worked out a nice little scam: He entered every auction, every time, so he could pass out coupons to female dominants who caught his eye.

Once the bidding ends, whoever won you is then obligated to enact your fantasy with you. You will usually retreat to a corner of the club together. Some clubs set a time limit on how long you are obliged to play; others let the players decide for themselves whether it'll last ten minutes or an eternity.

At all times, Dungeon Masters or safety monitors will keep an eye on you to be sure that whoever bought you does not violate their agreement to live out the fantasy. So, for example, if you put yourself up for sale as a foot slave who only wants to rub a woman's feet, the auctioneer will not sell you to anyone but a woman, and she will not proceed to tie you to a cross or anything else that wasn't in your description. You've entered a kind of mini-contract together, and both of you are expected to fulfill your side of the bargain.

Of course, if you get along wonderfully well, you can, by mutual consent, negotiate more than the scene you listed.

By the way, if you are bought by someone who is thinner, fatter, shorter, taller, or older than you were hoping for . . . that's too bad. You are obligated to follow through, according to the rules of this adult game.

If anyone breaks the terms of the auction (which the DJ usually announces right up front), the aggrieved party may report it to club management, who will have a talk with the violator or bounce them.

## BEFORE STEPPING OUT: A SHORT GUIDE TO SOCIAL ETIQUETTE

*I am a thirty-five-year-old submissive woman. I am planning to attend my first BDSM event next week. Part of me feels like a kid about to walk into a candy store! But another part is terrified that I'll make an idiot of myself. Is there some kind of etiquette I need to know? I'm also wondering whether I have to do SM with any dominant who asks. Do I have a right to turn them down, or will that seem rude?*

On the whole, SM clubs are safe, social environments where most people are friendly to newcomers. Naturally there will be some snobs and some introverts too, but you can count on finding at least a few people to make you feel welcome.

To ensure that you have a good experience, follow the rules in this guide.

### What to Wear, What to Wear?

Unless there is a stated dress code that specifies everyone must wear leather or fetish clothes, casual clothes (jeans) are perfectly acceptable. Avoid bright colors and pastels, leave your plastic pocket protectors at home, and just try to look your best.

If there is a dress code, don't buck it. The club will not make an exception for you. If you don't have the money for fetish clothes, wear black clothes and any black leather accessories (belts, shoes, vests, purses) you own. Other options include uniforms, army camouflage, undies, or lingerie and heels. And, yes, this fashion advice applies both to men and women. One tip: Men in lingerie will get a mixed reaction at best at a mostly gay leather gathering. So if you aren't sure of the club's conventions, stick to denim.

Expect to see people in all manners of dress. A lot of dominant men go for the black pants/black shirt look; dominant women often opt for a black jumpsuit or catsuit, or a black leather skirt or vest on top of black or dark clothes. But some people consider a trip to an SM event to be their version of Mardi Gras. You will see outrageous fetish outfits in rubber, latex, leather, and frills. I've seen everything from gents tightly clad, toe to scalp, in latex, to folks who walk around with clips and clamps and weights hanging off them like they were racks at a hardware store. Perhaps the most memorable was a fellow I saw in a unique combination of a bondage hood, a straight-jacket, pink anklets, and red high heels. Talk about a fashion statement!

You can also expect to see people in various states of undress. Full nudity is usually allowed at clubs that do not serve alcohol.

## Come Alone or Come with a Friend

This is not what you think it is.

It is acceptable for both men and women to enter a club or party alone. In my experience, the kinky crowds at SM clubs are far more polite than the party animals at regular bars. Aggressive come-ons are an absolute no-no at SM clubs and may be grounds for getting bounced.

Every SM event has staff appointed to monitor public safety. Security staff (also known as "Dungeon Masters") usually wear T-shirts to identify themselves and circulate through the crowd. They bounce people who get too loud or obnoxious. If some-one makes an untoward advance, tries to pressure you into a scene, doesn't respect your limits, or does anything else that goes against the rules and ethics of consensual kink, report it imme-diately to a Dungeon Master and he will quickly deal with it.

If the thought of going alone is too intimidating, and you don't have any friends who will accompany you, you'll need to contact one of your local SM membership organizations. Some sponsor trips to clubs or hold parties open to the public. You can stay with the group.

One bit of commonsense advice: Provide for your own transportation. Drive yourself there, if you can, or make sure before you go that there is safe, convenient public transporta-tion near the club. If you go with a group, make sure you have the number of a taxi service and the cash to pay for a car home. This way, if you want to cut out early you will not be depen-dent on people who think 2 A.M. means the night is still young.

## Amenities

SM clubs generally provide large-scale SM equipment (such as spanking benches, wooden crosses, bondage swings, and more) for public use. They are situated in various spots around the premises so that people have room to move. Some clubs will, on request, supply customers with small-scale equipment (such as spanking paddles or whips) as well.

Depending on the night and the club, once inside the door, you may see people frolicking with the equipment. Remember, it is all consensual play between adults. You will not see minors, violence, or unsafe sex.

As a courtesy to people who don't want to be seen on the street in fetish gear, clubs generally offer a coat check so you can change in their bathroom and leave your straight clothes at the door.

As noted earlier, SM clubs usually don't allow alcohol (or drugs) of any kind on the premises. If they do have a bar, chances are there will be restrictions on nudity. Most times, the only refreshments served are fruit juices or soft drinks. You won't be able to buy food, either, so eat before you go.

Don't expect a club to provide you with a partner or to keep a clutch of dominants or submissives on hand who are hungry to meet you. An SM club is not a dating or matchmaking service; it's a venue where kinky people can feel free to express their sexual identities without shame.

The only time you can be relatively certain of finding a partner is at a party hosted by a professional house of domination, where staff is on hand to facilitate the events. If you go to one, ask whether there is a fee for public scenes. There probably won't be, but it's better to ask first than to find out later that tickling someone's tootsies with your tongue just cost you $200.

## Hold Off Until You're Sure You're Ready

The first couple of times you go to an SM venue, I strongly recommend that you use your time to watch, listen, learn, and talk to the people around you. Even experienced players would do well to sit back until they have a good sense of the atmosphere of a new place.

I have known more than a few submissives who became so aroused by a first trip to an SM venue that they blithely agreed to do things they later regretted. They may have had a perfectly safe scene, which they explicited consented to act out. Indeed, they may have been the ones who approached the dominants and begged for it. What most novices don't realize, however, is that SM/fetish sex is not just physically intense. It is emotionally intense.

Monitors can protect you from other people. They can't protect you from your own hormones. Take the time to learn some of the social rituals and to get a sense of whether you like the atmosphere and the people. If you want to experiment, do it slowly, and let your partner know it's your first time. If you're worried they may reject you for being an "SM virgin," well, again, too bad: It is their right not to want to play with a novice.

I am one of those people who will not play with a novice at a club. I learned my lesson a dozen years ago when I was still fairly new to the Scene. An attractive submissive man followed me around for hours, begging me to give him the whipping he'd always dreamed of. I kept putting him off and putting him off—but eventually I melted and thought, "What the heck! He's a cutie! He knows what he's getting himself into!"

Wrong!

We had negotiated the scene and I respected his limits. But, to my astonishment—and then remorse—he dissolved into tears at the end. Sometimes a submissive will cry after SM simply from the sheer relief of letting go. Sometimes they just can't handle the intensity. In his case, I suspect he'd just been bottling up his feelings for a long time. Still, I ended up spending the rest of the evening holding a sobbing, incoherent, blubbering stranger in my arms and feeling like a heel.

Please learn from my mistake.

## Mind Your Kinky Manners

Never interrupt another person's scene. It's considered the height of rudeness. Maintain a respectful distance so they have room to play. Do not touch them, do not attempt to join in, and do not even talk to them until they are finished (unless they have explicitly invited you to join them). Players need to concentrate on what they are doing, so do not distract them.

Even after the scene is over, they may need privacy to cuddle or to talk quietly so the submissive can "come down" from the endorphin rush. Wait until they've moved away from the play area and rejoined the crowd before going over to them to say hello.

## Introductions

It is acceptable to walk up to people you don't know and to introduce yourself. It is not, however, acceptable to foist unwanted conversation on anyone or to pester them. If they send the signal that they are not interested in socializing with you, excuse yourself and move on.

(For a more comprehensive discussion of these basic concepts, read chapter 12, "The View from the Bottom: Sexual Submissives.")

## CHAPTER FIVE

# Erotic Bondage

### IS BONDAGE WRONG?

*Ever since I can remember, I've fantasized about being tied up by a powerful man and being treated like I have no choice but to give in to his sexual demands. I would never in reality want to be kidnapped or raped but these thoughts enter some of my fantasies too. I am only beginning to realize I am not the only one in the world who has them. Six months ago, I started dating my boyfriend. One day, he mentioned to me that he loved Betty Page and her funky old bondage poses. I decided to confess some of my fantasies to him. Since then, he has tied me up a number of times. I've loved it but there is still a part of me that feels ashamed of needing this. My boyfriend has tried to reassure me that it's okay because we both enjoy it and we aren't harming anyone, but I don't think it's as simple as that. Do you have any insights that will help me to understand why I need this? Am I wrong to give in to these needs?*

Without urging you to choose one way or another, I'll first say that your anxiety about bondage being wrong may have more to do with your fear that giving in to sexual pleasure is wrong, and not that there is actually something wrong with consensual bondage between adult partners.

Bondage is perhaps the single most common kinky sex fantasy. The idea of being tied up and helpless is frightening to some people for precisely the same reasons it's so erotic to others: Bondage makes a person physically vulnerable.

Looking at bondage fantasies from the outside, it's easy to understand why people find them scary. To the outsider, a bound human form looks demeaned and dehumanized and, even more shocking, it appears to be in immediate danger. Seeing someone restrained immediately summons images of victims whose lives are being threatened. All healthy creatures have a natural biological response to helplessness because (to oversimplify the science a bit) we are biologically programmed to interpret physical helplessness as a threat to our survival. So it's not surprising that a lot of people react to bondage with alarm, and think it is "sick" that people would enjoy it.

If you are one of the people who sees bondage as sick or unnatural, then it's important to remember that people who like to be tied up are not victims. They are lovers who have made an erotic agreement with their mates.

*Consent* is what distinguishes a bound victim you may see in a television report of a violent act and the bondage fans you may see in fetish magazines or at clubs. The person who is bound against her will by a criminal is terrified, unhappy, and in genuine danger. The misery she feels stands in direct contrast to the happiness a submissive feels when her lover ties her up. Someone who eroticizes bondage, and allows or asks a lover to tie her up, does so expecting pleasure and sexual satisfaction.

As someone who is more inclined to leap to a conclusion than to jump from a plane, I'm perpetually amazed by sky divers. It has never once occurred to me that plummeting to earth at high speed could be fun. Yet I've got close friends who can't get enough of such high-intensity sports, and I believe them when they say that these are physically and emotionally satisfying experiences for them. Despite my own slothful distaste for extreme sports, I can identify because I feel the same way about bondage and other types of high-intensity sex.

## WHAT MAKES BONDAGE SEXY?

*I've been with my lover for two years now. Since the beginning, he told me that he was very interested in bondage. I am an adventurous guy, and I have nothing against kink or SM, but it took a while for me to get comfortable with the idea. Now, after two years, and in light of the fact that we are getting ready to make a permanent commitment, I want to explore this with him. The problem is that although I'm emotionally ready, I still can't make the mental connection between sex and bondage. Can you help? What is it about being tied up that gets someone excited?*

Asking what makes a kinky activity feel so good to the kinky person doing it is like asking someone what makes dancing feel so good. It just does.

Not very satisfying, I know. But then, that is one of the problems with understanding other peoples' sexual quirks: If you don't share them, they just don't make much sense. We tend to go by our own experiences and preferences. At best, we can only take other peoples' word for it that an activity that may leave us shaking our heads in confusion has made them hot, moist, and happy.

Even though you may not share your lover's interest in bondage, or even understand why he or she would want that, the important thing is to work towards a compromise that meets both your needs, based on love and mutual respect.

To help you gain a perspective on the inner workings of why people enjoy being immobilized, here is a list of five common reasons people give to explain the joys of bondage.

## THE FIVE TOP REASONS WHY PEOPLE LOVE BONDAGE

### 1. The Freedom to Enjoy Sex

First, though it may seem paradoxical, erotic captivity makes the person who's tied up feel sexually freer. Bondage fans generally agree that one of the main attractions of bondage is that it allows them to embrace a more primal, sensual, and sexual being within themselves. Physical restraint relieves them of the normal mental restraints humans share—whether that is self-consciousness about our bodies, insecurity about our ability to satisfy our partners, guilt or shame about enjoying sex, or any of the other types of sex-related anxieties that inhibit us.

This is because the person who's tied up—powerless to cover himself, incapable of escape, and vulnerable to his partner's caresses—has surrendered sexual control to his partner. In surrender, he turns over the responsibility for his passionate responses to his partner. After all, if he's all tied up, it isn't his fault if he gets overly excited when his partner touches him. Without anxieties thwarting his responses, he may discover true erotic freedom through surrender.

From the dominant's side, the vulnerability and helplessness of the partner is erotic. A dominant feels a rush of pride and even some triumph in knowing that someone has surrendered control. Dominants often derive great pleasure from controlling all the partner's responses. The vision of a submissive in bondage alone turns many dominants on, for a wide variety of reasons. Perhaps the most common one is knowing that you can now "have your way" sexually with your partner.

## 2. Adrenaline Rush

Bondage, under any circumstances, is a physically and emotionally intense experience. It is the very essence of helplessness to be deprived the use of our limbs or to have our senses blocked. Even in a fully consensual setting, where the partners are long-time lovers, the bound person's body will go on full alert, reacting as if it were in danger.

She may have a faster heart and pulse rate; adrenaline and endorphins will likely flow. Even as these chemicals are unleashed, her brain begins compensating for the physical immobility by sending more information to other senses. For example, her sense of smell or taste may become sharper. Her skin may be more sensitive. A light caress or tickle that made her sigh before might cause her to squeal and writhe when she's tied up. Emotionally, she may experience fear, particularly at first, before she is aroused; endorphins may kick in and make her euphoric; some people run through hundreds of different emotions as the bondage continues; others relax so deeply they go into a near-trance of pleasure. Their eyes may glaze over, their eyelids may droop, their skin my grow flushed and radiant.

To return to my extreme sports analogy: You can think of bondage as a high-intensity sport for couch potatoes. Even though you may be tied to your lumpy old bed by the lumpy old person you've been married to for thirty lumpy years, your body may react to the situation as if you're a daredevil who has just stepped off a cliff with only a cord tied to your ankles to keep you from crashing into the abyss.

Yes, our brains aren't that smart: Even when we know we have consented to the bondage, our brain chemicals kick in and the intoxicating full-body high that results is precisely what so many people find appealing.

Although dominants may not experience quite the same endorphin rush, the feeling of power is its own intoxicant, and can bring on a state of euphoria too. I know from personal experience, for example, that doing bondage or other SM acts is a constantly reenergizing process: The energy I put out is more than doubled by the energy that comes back to me. I think this may help explain, for example, why dominants often can spend long hours doing complex, sometimes physically demanding scenarios without growing tired. The adrenaline rush keeps us very focused and energetic.

### 3. The Spiritual Journey

You may be surprised by this, but a growing number of kinky people believe there is a very definite connection between kinky sex and spirituality. You will find innumerable enclaves of pagans these days for whom SM acts (like bondage, piercings, or whippings) are a pathway to the divine. Pagans, though, are not the only ones who feel this way. Even firm believers in Judeo-Christian ideals report that they find spiritual elements in their bondage or SM play.

Part of the reason they give to explain this connection between spirituality and SM sexuality (with some folks even now calling SM "Sex Magick" or "Sexual Magic") is that high-intensity acts such as heavy bondage shut out the outside world and allow the bottom (or submissive) to take a journey within herself.

With a safe, expertly skilled top (or dominant), this journey can result in a state of complete tranquility and a feeling of oneness with God.

For dominants, the enjoyment comes from being able to provide this experience through one's own skill, sensitivity, and understanding of what the partner needs. Some dominants may enter that journey, deriving pleasure vicariously. Others feel spiritually rewarded in being able to provide the journey to their partners.

Using bondage to create a spiritual or meditative journey can also be seen as a service a dominant performs for the submissive. It embraces the concept of authority at a higher (in some cases shamanistic) level, in which taking responsibility for a partner's overall well-being is a chief virtue.

## 4. Dominance and Submission (D&S)

I will talk about the psychology of Dominance and Submission—from both male and female points of view—at much greater length later in the book. For now, though, I'll briefly explain D&S in the context of bondage.

For D&Sers, bondage is a blatant expression of their power relationships. Most (though not all) submissives react profoundly to bondage because it so vividly and unmistakably expresses their need to surrender power to their dominants. By granting their dominants the right to place them in a position of physical helplessness, submissives are symbolically stating that their trust in their dominant is absolute.

Dominants, meanwhile, are people who find it erotic to be in control. Bondage for them is a supreme example of their power over the submissive. Some find it sexy to elicit and control their partner's orgasms and devote most of their bondage play to teasing and pleasing. I've heard dominants describe it as being like a virtuoso musician who knows how to elicit the sweetest sounds from his precious violin.

When done safely, consensually, and with genuine caring, bondage builds ever-greater intimacy and trust between dominant and submissive partners.

## 5. Sadism and Masochism (SM)

Although I myself use the terms SM and D&S interchangeably, a lot of kinky people distinguish between them. For that reason,

I'll address the SM angle to bondage, which I didn't include in the D&S section just above.

There are people who do not think of themselves as dominant or submissive, but rather as people who pursue kinky sex for the physical sensations alone. Masochists, simply put, are people who need an intense level of stimulation to feel sexually satisfied. When it comes to bondage, then, they prefer pain and discomfort to snug, comfy bondage. They wish to be aware of their physical plight at every second. Even though they may transcend the pain, it is a vital part of the experience.

The masochist's counterpart in this is the sadist. Her pleasure may have nothing to do with caretaking and everything to do with consensually inflicting pain on a willing masochist.

Typical types of uncomfortable bondage includes hog-ties (where the bound wrists and bound ankles are joined together); rear hog-ties (same thing, only the limbs are pulled behind the back); suspension bondage (where the masochist may be hung by the wrists, ankles, or both); or bondage that doesn't necessarily immobilize them but which clamps and compresses them tightly. Corsetting and using nipple clamps, for example, would fall under the heading of compression bondage.

There are two heavier forms of bondage that are worth mentioning here. First is the ornate type of rope bondage which has developed as an erotic art for centuries among Oriental cultures (particularly the Japanese). With a special emphasis on aesthetics, this complex bondage takes many forms. At its most basic, it will consist merely of a few skillful knots, strategically arranged. At its most ornate, it includes weaving ropes so that the bound person appears suspended in a spider's web. Oriental bondage requires practice, a fair amount of skill, and a good aesthetic sense on the part of the dominant to achieve the right effect.

Perhaps the most misunderstood and visually alarming types of bondage are mummification and suspension. These types of bondage require an expert knowledge of safety issues.

In mummification, a person is completely encased, head to foot (whether in rubber, leather, bandages, Saran Wrap, or anything else), with only breathing holes (usually under the nose) left open. Even at its very lightest (using Saran Wrap, for example), mummification runs some risks, particularly if your partner has any preexisting medical conditions, is inclined to claustrophobia or panic, or is otherwise likely to have difficulty in a situation of total immobility.

In suspension, a person is raised up off the floor using any one of a variety of specialized equipment that can safely do this without injuring limbs or joints. Some typical types of suspension bondage include being raised by one's wrists, by one's ankles, by both ankles and wrists, and in a suspension device such as a "bondage swing."

Both mummification and suspension bondage are extremely intense. This type of play is not for inexperienced players. It is very easy to cause serious injury and even death if you don't know exactly what you are doing and if you don't use the proper equipment.

## PRISONERS OF LOVE

**Question:** *What do bondage fantasies, desert island sex fantasies, and naughty nurse fantasies have in common?*

**Answer:** The common denominator is captivity.

Many years ago, I met a young gentleman who had a fetish for iron fetters. He devoted much of his time (and income) to putting together a collection of iron restraints. I would see him clanking around merrily at clubs, his knapsack in one fettered hand, a glass of orange juice in the other (chained) one. His dream was to meet a nice girl who shared his fetish, so that the two of them could wear fetters together.

Since then, I've met people who have fetishes for an awesome range of restraints—from the garden-variety nipple clamps and penis harnesses one sees in adult toy shops, to extreme corsets, posture collars, bondage hoods, rubber suits, straightjackets, hospital restraints, orthopedic braces, and more.

Yet, for all that, not everyone who enjoys bondage cares about the particular type of equipment the dominant uses. What they seek is to live out their fantasies of being a helpless captive. Again, it's one of the fascinating contradictions of bondage that while the physical aspects are certainly very arousing, the emotional and sometimes spiritual aspects of surrender are what most bondage fans talk about.

Bondage enthusiasts, however, are not the only ones who fantasize about captivity. Captivity (or "conquest") fantasies are cited by sexologists as renowned as Masters and Johnson as the single most common adult sexual fantasy. Indeed, the variety of conquest fantasies is truly staggering. Below, I've organized captivity scenarios into five basic categories so you can understand their range.

Don't be surprised if you discover that, at some point in your life, your own fantasies may have ventured into one of them. In fact, don't be surprised if you have, at one time or another, ventured into all of them. The human imagination truly is limitless.

## THE FIVE TOP CAPTIVITY FANTASIES

### 1. Stranded Captivity

Fantasies in this category revolve around the basic premise of being helplessly stranded—whether it's on an island, in a desert or a jungle, or by magical transportation to another time zone or planet. You may be all alone or you may be trapped with other victims. Either way, at some point you are captured or conquered by either the local population or a predator in your midst. You may then be subjected to sexual assault or sexual pleasure, depending on whether your imagination runs to masochism or not.

### 2. Kidnapped Captivity

These fantasies revolve around a heart-stopping kidnapping scenario. The predators may be anonymous strangers (bikers often figure in a lot of Americans' fantasies) or someone you already lust after. In many of these fantasies, the kidnapped person is carried off, against his or her will. The setting could be a cabin in the woods, a luxurious estate on a mountaintop, a dank dungeon, or some other hideaway. Once there, the victim is sexually used by the kidnapper(s). Again, depending on the individual imagination, some fantasies will include torment and abuse, while others will imagine that the sex that ensues is exciting beyond his wildest dreams.

## 3. Prison Captivity

Although the common element in these fantasies, obviously, is being held behind bars, there are almost as many variations on this theme as on the ones above. People may fantasize about the simple hardships of prison life, from a poor diet, to the daily humiliations of public toilets and showers. Some people fantasize about being molested by guards or having their body cavities ruthlessly inspected. Prison fantasies include rape scenarios, verbal insults, interrogations, cruel physical punishments, and other hard-core types of abuse. There are also quite a few fetishists who are aroused by the equipment and accoutrements we associate with prisons and prison guards, most notably uniforms, handcuffs, fetters, heavy chains, and prison cells themselves.

Under this category you can also place a range of fantasies about being sent to boot camp and about police officers, law enforcement agents, and military personnel. Strange but true, there are people who don't just make a fetish of the uniforms but of the people who wear them. A few years ago, a woman in England who was arrested for shoplifting confessed that she wasn't a kleptomaniac, but a fetishist. She had hoped to get caught: Apparently, the entire drama of being arrested and handcuffed by the bobbies aroused her to the point of orgasm.

Needless to say, if your fantasies run along these lines, my advice is that you stick to consenting partners. You can find all the gear you need at a police-supply shop or military surplus store to get yourself arrested right in your own bedroom by someone you love. It will save you on legal bills.

## 4. Medical Captivity

In chapter 7 on fetishes, I'll talk about some of the specific types of medical equipment people eroticize. However, generally speaking, medical captivity involves fantasies about being confined to a bed or otherwise rendered helpless by some medically related condition.

Perhaps the most common and playful medical captivity fantasy is the "naughty nurse" scenario, where a sexy attendant takes advantage of the "patients" by seducing them. On the more extreme end, you'll find fantasies about distinctly unscientific "scientific" experiments by evil doctors, and sexual abuse by other patients or hospital staff.

There are dozens of fetishes associated with medical captivity. For example, people fantasize about orthopedic braces, plaster casts, bandages, wheelchair confinement, and traction. The daily rituals of hospital life also have a curious appeal. These include preoperative shaving of the genital or anal areas, getting enemas, using bedpans, rectal temperature-taking, gynecological or urological exams, catheterization, and all the other embarrassing, uncomfortable realities of hospital stays that make people feel vulnerable.

## 5. Sexual Captivity

Though most captivity fantasies involve some type of sex at some point, this set of fantasies centers around the idea of being held specifically and uniquely as a sex slave. The setting could be a harem or a brothel, a "sex farm," or even a monastery, or it could involve being tied up by a partner who then lets his or her "friends" take sexual advantage of the submissive.

A final note: Not all captivity fantasies involve force or coercion. In some cases, the person having the fantasy may see him- or herself as a willing volunteer or may perceive the person in charge as benevolent, and doing those terrible things because it's "for their own good."

A professional dominatrix once told me about a client who comes to her specifically to act out his fantasy of receiving an enema from a sympathetic nurse. The dominatrix wears a nurse's uniform, gently explains to him that the enema is important for his health, and then gently administers it, while reassuring him that though it may be embarrassing for him, it's necessary.

# BONDAGE TIPS AND TECHNIQUES

*My husband and I have been doing bondage since we got married six years ago. At first, I was surprised when he told me this was what he wanted in bed, but after seeing how much it excited him, I decided this was something I wanted to try too. Nowadays, we take turns getting tied up. We tie each other's arms and legs to the bedposts and then whoever is tied up gets oral sex (another reason I like being tied! ha!), and then we make love. Our sex is great but now we think we're ready to try for more variety. I see tips all the time on how to "spice up" lovemaking, but can you give us some creative ideas on how to spice up our bondage?*

I am just full of ideas.

Personally, I view bondage as an opportunity to enjoy a diverse range of scintillating erotic play. Although tying someone up is, in itself, arousing for me, what I really look forward to are all the ways I can tease and erotically torment my bound partner.

Although many couples use bondage primarily as foreplay, I recommend you think of bondage not merely as a way to get someone ready for intercourse, but as a legitimate form of sexual intimacy, whether or not it is followed by conventional lovemaking. Or, as philosophers and poets have long advised—though generally with a more flowery vocabulary—enjoy the trip and don't worry about the destination.

In the following practical guide, I offer you a long list of options for making the most of your bondage sessions.


## CLAMPS, CUFFS, AND CROSSES:
## A BASIC GUIDE TO BONDAGE TOYS

The number of bondage devices that people use and have used throughout history could fill an encyclopedia. It would be impossible to list them all here. Over the centuries, creative minds around the globe have fashioned thousands, if not millions, of different appliances to immobilize, restrict, compress, and otherwise impose control over a person's body. Historically, all too many of these devices were used cruelly, on prisoners and victims. In this book, I concentrate uniquely on safe, mutually consensual bondage, done for pleasure.

Below, I list the most basic types of devices and toys that lovers enjoy. Included in this list are a number of things (such as blindfolds, gags, chastity belts, and clamps) that are not used specifically to tie someone up, but to add to their helplessness, increase their stimulation, or deprive them of certain senses ("sensory deprivation") or functions.

Sensory deprivation is not an element in all bondage fantasies, but most experienced people will at least have experimented with items (such as blindfolds) that limit sensory input and output. The basic idea behind sensory deprivation is that, by not letting the tied-up person receive information through the normal channels (eyes, ears, mouth), their sensitivity to physical stimulation rises, as does their ability to focus intently on the bondage experience.

For most equipment, I describe the styles and construction materials you are likely to find at a reasonably well-stocked adult toy store. Please remember, though, that many of these devices are crafted by independent artisans who interpret their designs differently. (Indeed, the mark of an accomplished kinky craftsperson is that he or she will wring some new changes on standard old designs.) Where I've described something as made of leather, you may find that your local craftsperson selected to work in chain mail, rubber, or any of a number of other materials.

As I said, I won't attempt a catalogue of every type of bondage equipment here. Instead, this is a solid introduction to all the basic bondage and sensory-deprivation toys that kinky people use to heighten their sexual pleasure.

## Head

The range of bondage toys that are placed on the head range from the very mild (such as soft, fleecy night masks used as blindfolds) to the extreme (full-head bondage hoods). You can also find "head harnesses," a series of leather straps, riveted together, with buckle fasteners, and often including built-in leather bits (gags) and blindfolds. I recommend the type where these accessories can be easily snapped out. "Head cages" are far rarer and also more extreme: There are steel varieties that consist of strips welded together to form a cage in the shape of the head (these metal cages are also known as "branks"). There are wooden ones as well, usually carved boxes that provide enough space for the head and neck to fit comfortably.

Head cages are for more experienced players. Although they are not dangerous, their effect on the submissive can be radical: Covering up the head is an intensely emotional experience, and can easily cause claustrophobia or a panic attack in an inexperienced submissive.

Slightly kinder, though still for heavy players, are the full-head hoods. Usually made of leather, with openings for the eyes, mouth, and nose (so the person can breathe freely), these are still powerful and severe, but not quite as restrictive as the cages. Some hoods have snap-on blindfolds and gags; others have zippers over the eyes and mouth.

For novices who want to experiment with some type of a hood, I suggest you start at the very mildest level—the footsie end of panty hose, pulled down over your head, will give the budget-conscious a taste of this type of restriction. Another very safe option is a simple wool ski mask. And, if you insist on investing in this type of play, check out some of the soft, stretchy fabric hoods available at most bondage boutiques.

I hope I don't have you tell you this, but I will anyway: Never, ever put plastic, or any other fabric or material that isn't porous, over nostrils and mouth at the same time. The results could be fatal.

*Eyes:* Blindfolds are another common sensory-deprivation toy. Though they come in different materials and different colors, most commercially available blindfolds are made in essentially the same style: a mask that fits over the eyes and has either thin elastic or straps with buckles to hold the mask in place.

For the novice, an inexpensive sleeping mask, which you can find at any pharmacy, is adequate. You can also use a scarf or bandanna, leaving a flap in the front and tying the ends behind the person's head.

If you want something that looks a little more intimidating, opt for a soft leather blindfold with a buckle closure. For a safe, secure fit, I'd recommend one with a thick, fleecy or softly padded lining that cushions the eyes and reduces any risk of putting pressure on the optic nerve.

The most important thing to remember about blindfolds is that, as harmless as they seem, even the lightest-weight one can cause damage to the eye if you tie it on too tight. Secure a blindfold only tight enough to block the person's vision and ask them to tell you if there's any pressure on their eyeballs. If there is, loosen the blindfold and adjust it accordingly.

*Ears:* Another sensory-deprivation embellishment during bondage is to control hearing. There are basically two popular ways of doing this. This first is by using simple earplugs. Don't just stick cotton balls in your (or your partner's) ears. Use real earplugs, which are engineered to block the delicate ear canal safely and effectively. Music stores and gun shops carry the most effective types.

The other way dominants may control their partners' hearing is by putting them in headphones. I've known people who have their partners go through an entire bondage experience listening to gentle classical music, and others who make their own tapes, selecting songs and snatches of narrative all intended to heighten the mood.

*Mouth:* Gags are used to stifle speech and muffle noise. People's opinion of gags vary. Some find them a bit too stringent, others can't imagine bondage without them. The most common commercially available type are the "ball gags," brightly colored rubber balls threaded on a leather lanyard, whose ends you tie behind the person's head.

You may feel otherwise, but ball gags aren't my favorite. They force a partner's mouth very wide, which can strain the jaw (particularly if your partner is small-boned). Jaw strain just isn't sexy and is potentially harmful. Second, they are messy. A gag can cause a person to drool and salivate heavily, especially when their jaws are pulled wide—plus, the soft ball tends to get chewed up a bit, so it's just not the most hygienic option.

My own favorite is a small, soft leather bit (about two inches), which the submissive can chew without destroying, and which fits neatly inside the mouth, reducing the drool factor. It is just as effective as a ball gag in muffling noises. Also, the leather has much more give than a rubber ball, so the potential for jaw strain is greatly reduced.

If you're new to gags, don't bother with the commercially produced kind until you know for sure it's something your partner enjoys. Instead, experiment with a cotton scarf or bandanna or a pair of undies. Absolutely never stick a gag in someone's mouth so deep that they begin to choke, splutter, or give any other signs of distress.

Do not tie the gag tightly. Unless you want to cause discomfort, tying it tightly just puts strain on your partner's jaw. If you want the gag to have a bit more oomph, tie a knot or two in the middle of the scarf and gently fit the knot inside your partner's mouth before tying the ends.

*Neck:* Collars are one of the basic pieces of bondage equipment that people collect. In fact, collars have become so popular that a ritual has grown up around them. "Collaring" refers to the formal, often public, commitment ceremony between dominant and submissive. At that time, the dominant will place his or her collar on the submissive, who then vows permanent obedience.

Collars don't always figure into actual erotic play. Instead, it is their symbolism that people find erotic. For this reason, although the most common types of collars are either a length of metal chain (secured by a steel lock, which the dominant keeps) or a leather collar that buckles in the back (with or without rings for locks), some couples opt for alternatives such as high-quality gold chain necklaces, which pass as ordinary jewelry. The reason for this is that the submissive can discreetly wear the collar twenty-four hours a day without attracting strange looks from coworkers and friends.

There are collars, however, that are expressly designed to fit into bondage play. These include "posture collars" (wide, stiff-leather collars that force the submissive to keep his or her head high) and steel-reinforced (or full-metal) collars with rings, which can be attached to other bondage devices.

By the way, one of the common faux pas that novice dominants make is to wear collars as a fashion statement. Traditionalists scoff at this, since, as I just said, collars symbolize slavery or submission. Personally, I am not the biggest stickler for tradition, believing as I do that if it turns you on, that's good enough. Still, in this case, I have to agree: The only fashion statement that a dominant makes when she wears a collar is that she is clueless.

## Arms/Hands

The bondage device most commonly associated with kinky sex is the humble pair of handcuffs. Actually, the cheap metal handcuffs sold as novelty items in adult sex boutiques are the worst to use because they are the least comfortable and the most likely to break. Handcuff aficionados invest a little more money and buy genuine police/military handcuffs, which offer heavier restraint but slightly more comfortable wear, or steel fetters.

The enormous popularity of bondage as a sensual variation on lovemaking has given rise to an enormous range of inexpensive, lightweight cuffs intended primarily for the sensual experience of bondage, and not for serious restraint. You can find sets of matching wrist and ankle cuffs in satin, soft leather, and fake fur, some with Velcro closures. For more serious bondage play, some people prefer thickly cushioned, self-belted leather cuffs. Some are lined with fleece, others are padded with leather, and most have metal rings on the outside so the cuffs can be attached to other bondage devices or tied off to bedposts.

Although more difficult to obtain, hospital restraints are also very popular, partly because of the medical twist, but also because they offer comfort, quality, and security for those interested in extended bondage scenarios.

Esoteric but quite sensual are bondage mittens. A common mitten design includes belts at the wrists and metal rings at the tips so that the mitten can be attached to other devices. A stringent version of the bondage mitten is the bondage arm-glove—one enormous glove that may be worn in front or back: The hands and arms are inserted and belts or laces are adjusted, forcing the arms together. When worn in back, the chest is thrust forward by the large glove pulling the arms backwards.

## Nipples

Nipple clamps (or clips) are the most popular items you will find in the kinky section of adult toy stores. Although the basic style is a metal spring-action clip with rubber insulation at the ends to protect the skin, you will find dozens of variations on this theme, plus many other styles that do not rely on springs, but have screw mechanisms, adjusting rings, and other tension-controlling devices. Most clamps that you can purchase commercially are connected by a metal chain.

If you're just starting out, select small, lightweight clamps, heavily insulated at the ends, with lightweight chains and either a screw or ring to adjust tension. Make sure there is a reliable tension-adjustment mechanism. If you already have experience with them, you have a lot of different options for increasing the sensation. You can find heavy clamps with tight spring mechanisms, weighted clamps, big clamps with big chains, and weights that can be hung from the chain to add a tugging sensation to the clamping.

Generic clothespins are a cheap alternative favored by kinky folks. The wooden kind work just fine and, if you've got any manual skills, you can always drill tiny holes in the ends and connect them yourself with string or thin chain. The truly diabolical may even connect a long series of clothespins on string, attach them individually to sensitive flesh, then tear them off with one excruciating yank. This is called a "zipper."

## Genitals

Not surprisingly, because they protrude, and because submissive men so enjoy the terror and pain of having their genitals handled roughly, there is a whole cottage industry devoted to devices to restrain and deliver sensation to male genitalia. Female genitalia do not lend themselves very well to bondage devices. Most bondage fans rely on threading ropes, straps, or chains between female partners' legs to separate the labia or to create harnesses around them for various types of bondage play.

*Rings:* If you've ever browsed through an adult toy store or catalogue, you've undoubtedly seen "cock rings." These are generally made of steel, rubber, or leather.

There are several basic styles of cock ring. The most common is a simple ring of steel that slides over the penis and is worn at the base, on the assumption that when the penis is erect, the shaft will fill out the ring and the ring will stem further blood flow. Other types encircle the penis and the testicles. Some people claim it helps them to maintain an erection, others say it keeps them erect without letting them orgasm, and others just like the extra sensation of something gripping their organs. There are also adjustable rings made of leather, and with snaps.

Not all rings are created equal. Just as there's variation in the size of men's organs, so too will you find rings of all sizes for men of all sizes. This is the obvious advantage of purchasing an adjustable leather ring, although some people don't get the rigid tightness they enjoy in a steel ring. Rubber is another alternative—not as inflexible as steel but still rigid enough to squeeze the shaft tightly.

You may also see very large rings or exotic-looking ones with two or three rings soldered together. The large ones are not meant for Goliaths (alas!): They are meant to go around both the base of penis and the testicles.

*Cages and Harnesses:* There are so many different appurtenances that could be labeled "cages" or "harnesses" that I'll only describe the most common ones. Generally speaking, cages and harnesses enforce chastity because they either restrict erections or enclose the penis in a device that makes penetration difficult or impossible.

The most common type resemble little steel cages but are shaped to accommodate the shaft of the penis. They are typically a series of rings, in graduated sizes (narrower on top, wider on the bottom), connected on either side by metal strips so the "cage" is rigid. It usually attaches to the genitals by means of a leather strap (with a buckle) that is fastened around the testicles.

The "Gates of Hell" is a similar device: a series of rings, but this time connected only on one side, usually by a strip of hard leather. The extra flexibility doesn't make it less severe: The rings themselves are usually tighter than in a cage, which means greater restriction of blood flow to the penis.

A "cock harness" is a kinder variation on the cage, and is usually made of stiff leather, with snaps or buckles to adjust the tightness. The general design will include a thick ring of leather (a few inches wide) for the penis, plus an adjustable leather strap that adjusts under and around the testicles. A harness will also often have some kind of metal ring on it to which a bondage device may be attached. For example, a rope or chain may be run through the ring and then tied to a collar or to a piece of equipment (to keep the person from moving). Dominants also may clip a leash to the ring and lead their partner around by their genitals—something that certainly makes a statement when you're out at an SM party.

*Butterfly Board:* One of the more intense genital punishment devices, this is a thin wood board with a circular hole carved out, just large enough to squeeze the genitals through. The man remains on one side, his genitals are pushed through to the other, and the top will then insert small, sterile needles into the loose skin of his scrotum, securing the sac to the board. Ouchie. Not for pain wimps.

*Gloves:* A penis or genital glove is a leather pouch in the shape of male genitals. The most common model has a pouch for the scrotum and a leather cylinder for the penis, with laces on the side to adjust the glove as tightly as one wishes. Generally, the casing for the shaft is complete but in some models there is an opening at the end so that the glans remains exposed and vulnerable to other types of teasing or punishment.

The most sensual variety will be made of soft leather, and its main purpose is to encase the genitals comfortably while delivering the feeling of control (or chastity). However, there are more stringent versions, designed for people who like CBT. Some gloves are constructed so that when the laces are tightened, the testicles are forced down and away from the penis, creating tension and adding sensation. There are also models that feature tiny spikes on the inside of the scrotal pouch— when the glove is tightened, these prick the skin rather uncomfortably.

*Parachutes/Weights:* Another means of delivering intense sensations to the male genitals is by stretching the testicles away from the penis. One method is by using a glove, but a more direct and extreme way is with a "parachute." This is a circular band of leather designed to fit around the base of the testicles—when adjusted in place, it looks somewhat like the man is wearing a tiny clown collar around his balls.

The leather is punched with a few holes, from which thin chains hang. The chains are used for weights that will pull down on the testicles. If you've ever seen fishing-line weights in adult toy shops and wondered what they were for, they are *not* made for an afternoon on Walden Pond. The heavier the weight, the more intense the sensation and also the more careful you must be. Unless you like the herniated look, be very careful or you will cause damage if you try to stretch the scrotum too quickly.

*Genital Clamps:* Some of the same types of clips used on nipples may also be used on genitalia, both male and female. The only really safe place to use clamps on a man is on the skin of his scrotum: With the exception of clothespins (which work very nicely on women as well), most clipping and clamping devices are too intense to place on the penis and could cause unwanted damage. Vaginal lips, however, are a bit sturdier and even heavy clamps can be used on them, particularly if the tips are well insulated with rubber. The main problem that arises using clamps on the labia is that lubrication from arousal may cause the clamps to slide right off.

*Chastity Belts:* These are equal-opportunity genital restraints because there are models available for women as well as for men.

Obviously, the design features for each sex are different. A male chastity belt will usually have a built-in restraint to accommodate the penis. Depending on the level of control and humiliation desired, the belt may also include a butt plug. A woman's chastity belt too may feature a butt plug in the rear, and may also have a built-in dildo to block the vagina. However, most models simply block the vagina so that entry by a penis (or hand) is impossible, but leave just enough space to allow urination. In both cases, extended use of a butt plug or a dildo can cause problems, so these are generally only for shorter-term wear.

The most popular type of chastity belts commercially available are engineered of lightweight stainless steel and can be worn fairly comfortably for long periods of time. Only one word of caution: Be careful when traveling. I heard some years ago of a man who actually triggered an airport security alarm with his chastity belt, and it took a whole lot of explaining (and a good deal of embarrassment, since he was required to strip) before he was able to board his flight. Unless your thirst for humiliation knows no end, I suggest you keep this possibility in mind.

**Legs**

There are several key pieces of equipment designed to restrain feet and legs. The most common by far are ankle cuffs, which are large-sized metal handcuffs with a length of chain connecting the cuffs. Leather cuffs and fetters are popular too. Another very popular item is the "leg-spreader," an adjustable, rigid bar (usually made of metal, but also wood) with cuffs (typically made of leather) on either end. Ankles are secured in the cuffs and the bar is adjusted to the desired spread (usually between three and four feet). This places the bound partner in a position of extreme vulnerability, because his or her thighs are forced wide apart, leaving the genitals helplessly exposed.

Other common leg/foot restraints include "thigh to wrist restraints," which are wide belts that buckle around the thighs, with leather wrist cuffs (also belted) riveted to them so that each wrist may be secured to the outside of each thigh. There are also "thumb cuffs," which may be used either on thumbs or on the big toes of feet. These resemble miniature metal hand-cuffs but feature solid-body construction.

## A Note About Budget Bondage

Creative bondage fans like to browse through hardware stores, office-supply stores, medical-supply catalogues, and crafts catalogues, and patronize merchants you wouldn't normally think of as purveyors of bondage toys. You'd be surprised how many ordinary objects can be used in a kinky context.

Hardware stores are a particular favorite of perverts. You can find lots of unusual clamps and vise-like gadgets there—not to mention lifetime supplies of ropes, chains, and locks. Medical-supply places and craft shops also sell devices for clamping or holding things in place. Personally, I've always found that kitchenware shops are a cornucopia for the creative pervert. Put another way: spatulas, wooden spoons, and wire whisks, OH MY!

The only warning here is that if you do buy something not intended to be used as you plan to use it, make sure to test it carefully for safety first—but you already knew that, right?

### FIFTEEN WAYS TO TEASE YOUR TIED-UP LOVER

1. Use a feather to gently explore every nook and cranny of your partner's body. Special areas to focus on: thighs; the lower belly and fleshy areas surrounding the genitals, breasts, and nipples; underarms; backs of knees and insides of elbows; wrists; hands and fingers (including the webs between fingers); back of the neck; the face (trace your partner's hairline, nose, lips, eyelids, and eyebrows, then trace a line down to the neck); soles of the feet. If the bondage permits it (for example, if the person is tied spread-eagle), draw the feather up between their legs and tease them both front and back.

2. Take a little scrap of fur or fleece and rub it lightly over your partner's sensitive areas: thighs, belly, soles, breasts, nipples, neck, and so on. Lay the fur against your partner's face so he or

she can smell it and feel it brush against his or her lips. Rub it against your partner's genitals too, gently squeezing and massaging the area. If you oppose the use of animal fur, use faux fur.

3. Take a silk or satin scarf and run it over his or her body. You can wrap it lightly around her breasts or his penis, or loop it around thighs, and then slowly, gently pull it loose again, making sure the silk caresses his or her genitals as you pull. Push the edge of the scarf into your partner's mouth, just far enough inside so your partner can taste it, then slowly pull it out again. (You may do the same to other orifices, of course.) You might wish to add a drop or two of your perfume or cologne to the scarf. Better still, while your partner watches, run the scarf over your own genitals or other sexy body parts before using it on your partner: This will enhance your intimacy a notch.

4. Alternate hot and cold sensations. One of the sexiest ways to do this is to have a hot beverage (coffee or tea) and a cold one (any iced drink will do) at hand. Take a few sips of the hot beverage and then let your warmed lips and tongue explore your lover's body, then switch to the iced drink and do the same.

5. Make it real hot. Using a pure white candle (or any candle that does not contain dyes, which can burn the skin), raise the candle at enough of a distance from your partner's body so that you can let the wax drip onto him or her without causing any burns. The effect you want is intense warmth. You know how parents check a baby's bathwater? Do the same here by trying it out on yourself first. Holding the candle in one hand and as far as you can away from yourself, let a few drops of hot wax fall onto your skin. Gradually bring the candle closer until the wax feels very warm. Practice until you are sure you know how to do this without causing any burns.

6. Make it real cold. Take an ice cube and run it over your partner's body, tracing lines, following curves, slipping it into orifices. You can use the edge for tight spots and the flat side of the cube for wider surfaces.

7. Try a little cootchie-cootchie-coo. Some people will find tickling unbearable, but others may find it unbearably erotic. So

use your common sense and don't keep doing this to someone who really loathes it. But tickling can be a delicious torment to someone who is bound. You don't need to dig your fingers deep into their ribs. Instead, begin lightly and gently tickling the soles of their feet, their belly button, their neck and underarms, and so on. Make sure to let your partner catch his or her breath from time to time. Stop when and if your partner lets you know that the sensation is more than he or she can stand. You aren't hurting them, but extreme tickling can be very cruel in its own way, so proceed cautiously.

8. If you and your partner enjoy oral sex, bondage presents a multitude of opportunities for your mutual pleasure. You can use your tongue, lips, and teeth as boldly and creatively as you like. You don't have to limit the oral explorations just to his genitalia, but can enjoy your partner's body with your mouth, the way you might savor a fine meal. Alternate types of oral caresses: flick your tongue against his nipples, dab it into his ears, give him wet sucking kisses on his thighs.

You can also receive oral pleasures from your partner. For example, you can carefully position yourself over him, inserting your nipples into his mouth and thus "forcing" him to suck them. You can squat above his head and lower yourself down (being careful not to smother the poor thing!), and have your partner lick and kiss your genitals. Indeed, if you are reasonably fit, you can slowly and gently bring any and every area of your body—from your fingers to your toes—close to your partner's lips for oral stimulation. If you are physically challenged, consider changing the type of bondage: Instead of having your partner tied to the bed, bind his wrists and his ankles so that you can move him around on the bed. (Or simply tell him what you want, and let him wriggle around and try to reach those places on your body by himself. Sometimes the struggling alone can be erotic.)

9. Biting and scratching can be very pleasurable, but unless you already know your partner is a heavy masochist, start out very gently—nibbling here and there, raking your fingernails across his or her flesh (but without leaving scratch marks). You can build the intensity over time, if it's something you both

enjoy, but always start out slowly and see how much sensation your partner can eroticize.

10. One of my own personal favorite ways of teasing and tormenting someone in bondage doesn't involve the use of implements. Instead, I like to talk to him, and say things which make his brain reel a bit. For example, after I have someone tied up, I like to talk about how helpless he looks and how helpless he must feel to be all tied up. I might challenge him to try to escape by struggling against the ropes (or chains or whatever I've used). When he struggles and fails to escape, it will only reinforce his helplessness and his excitement. I might point out that, trussed up as he is, I could do literally anything to him that I wanted. I might mention, for example, that I could use him as a sex toy for my own pleasure. Perhaps I will take my pleasure from him, orally or vaginally. Or I might threaten him with the possibility that I will leave him this way for a while, and not allow him to have an orgasm until I am ready—if I'm ever ready. Kind of mean, aren't I?

11. Another way to tease someone is to let them watch as you slowly undress. Knowing that you are only inches away from them, but that they are helpless to touch you, will make them squirm with desire. If you're the exhibitionistic type, you can do a full striptease, music and all.

12. Keep them on the edge of orgasm by directly stimulating their genitals (or other erogenous zones you know will bring them to climax), and then stopping when they seem ready to climax. While you keep your frustrated partner waiting (and hoping and begging) for release, you can try any of the techniques I describe above.

13. A slightly more torturous (or pleasurable, depending on your partner) variation on this is to repeatedly bring your partner to climax. Your partner will feel that he or she is being "forced to cum" (a very exciting fantasy for people who enjoy bondage). Submissive men often fantasize about being "milked"—i.e., having their genitals manipulated repeatedly. This fantasy also contains an element of masochism as continual manipulation like this will eventually cause them serious dis-

comfort. On the other hand, submissive women (particularly those with nearly unlimited abilities to orgasm) may find this a delightful "punishment." Just be aware that your partner's mileage will vary, and that one submissive's pleasure could be another's punishment.

The following techniques are aimed at more experienced people, and should only be done with a partner's clear *advance* consent.

14. People who identify as sadomasochists enjoy combining intense stimulation with bondage. So, for example, if the one being tied up enjoys clamping, pinching, whipping, or any other extreme sensations, the person who's tied them can take advantage of their bound helplessness to deliver such painful pleasures. If the bound person is a masochist, you can add to their excitement by attaching clips and clamps to nipples, breasts, labia, scrotum, thighs, and other sensitive areas. Be aware that people who you think are completely immobilized may sometimes surprise you with a burst of adrenaline-driven strength and suddenly lurch or seem actually to leap within their bounds.

For this reason, a top should be careful in the choice of punishment implements. Do not use sharp tools unless you are sure the bottom cannot jump and be cut or pierced accidentally. You are safest sticking to small, simple slapping devices which won't significantly harm anyone even if the blow falls in the wrong place. You're safer still if you just use your hands. Remember that a person in bondage usually experiences things more intensely, so a little goes a long way. Well-placed pinches, cruel twisting of soft flesh, and hard squeezes of sensitive areas will keep most masochists moaning with pleasure.

15. How about a nice smooth shave? Shaving off a partner's body hair can be fantastically erotic. Unless you are an expert with the straight razor, stick to a safety razor. Don't use an electric shaver—long body hairs will catch in the blades and get pulled, causing pain. If your partner is extremely hairy, you might want to trim in advance, very carefully, either with small scissors (haircutters are good) or with an electric beard/mustache trimmer.

Personally, I prefer a safety razor: It gets the job done cleanly and with the lowest risk of accidental cuts or nicks. Prepare a bowl of warm, soapy water, or get a good shaving cream that will moisturize the skin. Make sure you have water (running or in a bowl) so you can rinse off the safety blade as you work.

Depending on what you and your partner have discussed or negotiated, you may choose only to shave the genitals or you can be more adventurous and shave any leg or chest hair. Most submissives find it the height of helplessness to watch as the dominant slowly removes hair from their body.

Do it sensuously. Do *not* rush. Remind your submissive to hold very still. If your partner squirms a lot, you risk nicking them. Stop and wait until they calm down and tell them again that you can only do this if they lie still. If they are unable to do so, stop. Unless the person is extraordinarily ticklish, the only physical sensation they should feel during a shaving is pleasure.

Again, I will emphasize that you should get advance consent for this scene. Don't wait until his legs are shaved to discover that your male lover is playing tennis with his boss the next day. Similarly, make sure your female lover isn't about to visit the gynecologist just when you've come up with the nifty idea of shaving her pubes bare. Obviously, if your partner would find any of the above wickedly erotic, that's fine—just don't put anyone in a situation that can cause emotional distress.

Finally, a little aftercare will keep the skin healthy and rash-free. Apply (or have your partner apply) a moisturizing cream to the shaved areas. An over-the-counter cortisone preparation is especially good. This will help prevent razor bumps, itchiness, and rashes that are common after shaving sensitive skin. Keep applying the creams daily until the hair grows back or the shaved skin remains clear for several days.

## BONDAGE NEVERS

### If You're the One Who Is Tied Up . . .

• Never drink alcohol or do drugs before you get tied up. Intoxicants alter your perceptions of sensation, and dull your capacity to judge whether the bondage is just enough or way too much. If you can't do the bondage without getting high first, then do not do the bondage.

• Never let someone you don't know really well put you in bondage that you can't easily escape. Don't believe what anyone may tell you over the Internet, at a party, or during a brief encounter—psychopaths are accomplished liars. Once you let someone tie you up, you are putting yourself at their mercy. Make sure they have *mercy* before you hand over control of your life to them. Get to know the person first, find out if someone else knows them and thinks they're trustworthy, and always start out with light types of bondage you can get out of should the person start acting wacky. (I recommend this even to men who visit professional dominatrices: You *must* have solid reasons to believe that someone is reliable before you put your life into their hands. Again, any nut can take out an ad claiming to be a domme, so caveat emptor.)

• Never conceal health or psychological issues of any kind. Do you have asthma? Arthritis? Diabetes? Irritable bowel syndrome or another condition that requires that you have immediate access to the toilet? Are you phobic about blindfolds? Are you claustrophobic? Before you allow someone to put you in bondage, talk to them, in depth, about any physical or emotional challenges you may have, and make sure they not only understand your limits but will respect them unquestioningly.

• Never get so carried away by the experience that you lose all sense of what's going on with your own body. Many people experience an ecstatic trance during bondage. That's lovely, but please don't enter the ecstasy so completely that you ignore the fact that your nipples have been numb for an hour.

If you've ever done hatha yoga, you know that some of the exercises are designed to enhance awareness of each part of the body. A person in bondage should try to do the same by mentally checking their body state. Every so often, while you are bound, review your situation. Are your nipples, hands, feet, or any other body part getting numb? Are you finding it difficult to breathe? Are you getting muscle spasms? Is an old injury starting to hurt? Do you feel faint or nauseous? The moment you sense that something isn't quite right, let your partner know so he or she can release you immediately.

## If You're the One Doing the Tying . . .

• Never drink alcohol or do drugs before you tie someone up. Nothing hurts a dominant's judgment more than intoxicants. They make you unsteady, less mentally aware, and less emotionally caring. If you can't tie someone up without getting high first, then do not tie them up.

• Never panic. If the person you tied up exhibits behavior that frightens you—whether it is excessive struggling or writhing, screaming, hyperventilation, or any other dramatic behavior you can't cope with—proceed calmly to release them in as quick and efficient a manner as humanly possible. If you panic, you may make a dumb mistake, and a dumb mistake in bondage can cause serious injury. If you know already that you have a tendency to panic or to bolt away when a crisis arises, then bondage is definitely not for you.

• Never leave someone in rigid bondage alone. When you put a person in a helpless situation, you take on the job of monitoring his or her health. It is your responsibility to ensure that the bondage remains a safe, pleasurable experience for your partner. Monitor your bondees frequently, checking their limbs, watching their reactions, and making sure that they are breathing regularly (and not hyperventilating, which could lead to dizziness and fainting). Ask them periodically if they feel okay—if they are gagged, prearrange signals they can use (like wiggling a finger or a foot) to say yes and no. If you must leave the room for a few minutes, remove any gags and make sure you can hear your partner should he or she call for assistance.

• Never restrain someone unless you have the means to free them instantly should an emergency arise. If you're using ropes, keep a pair of heavy scissors or a good-quality knife at hand so you can quickly cut them loose. The same goes for other types of soft bondage, such as panty hose, Saran Wrap, latex sheeting, and so on.

Always have the appropriate cutting tool handy so you can quickly and safely release your partner. If an emergency finds you frantically searching for that pair of nail clippers you know you stuck in a drawer somewhere, your partner is in big trouble.

If you use a knife, make sure you place the blunt edge of the knife against your partner's skin under the ropes, then pull the blade upward, cutting as you go. Do not cut down, or slice at the material from different directions. Never let the blade touch your partner's skin during an emergency.

If you are using metal cuffs, fetters, or locks, make sure you know exactly which keys go to which device and place the keys in easy reach, neatly organized, so you can use them in a hurry. It's a good idea to practice locking and unlocking the devices by yourself before locking anyone into them. Not only will you look stupid if you fumble with keys, but it will take you longer to get your partner out of the bondage.

If you do suspension bondage, use "panic snaps"—quick-release snaps that can be sprung without loosening tension on the line (so you don't have to lift the person to release them). You can buy these at any good hardware store.

• Never leave a person in a device that restricts their breathing.

• Never leave a person in stringent bondage for long periods of time until you are completely familiar with their reactions and their level of tolerance.

• Never tie a blindfold very tightly. You can cause damage to the eyes if you press on them too hard. Tie a blindfold on just securely enough so your partner can't see. If you're just starting out with bondage, I recommend you purchase a soft, fleecy sleeping mask, with a thin elastic band that goes around the head. It will get the job done with low to no risk of harm.

• Never tie a gag too tight. This mainly applies to ball gags and gags with rubber or leather inserts that fit inside the mouth. When you keep a person's mouth open by use of a gag, saliva will begin to collect. They may drool a little. Watch the drool. The could begin to choke on it. Some people might get queasy from the gag. Again, make sure they can communicate with you using a nonverbal signal, so you know the instant the gag starts causing problems.

• Never leave clamps on someone's body for too long and always make sure to test them on yourself first to see how tight they are. (You don't need to put them on your own nipples: Clip them on the web of skin between your thumb and forefinger.) If you use tight clamps, be aware that if you leave them on for more than ten to fifteen minutes at a time, your partner's nipples may begin to get numb. Numbness means the clamps must come off. It is a warning signal that the nerves are being stressed and that damage will soon develop.

I have heard depressing stories of clueless dominants who foolishly leave clips and clamps on a partner's body for hours at a time, even overnight (!), and then can't understand why the nipples are never as sensitive again.

Start your partner out with lightweight clamps, and leave them on for short periods of time. After a while, you'll be able to move up the nipple clip food chain and use heavier, more vicious ones (if that's what you both like). Check periodically to find out if there is any numbness. It's a good idea to remove them every ten or fifteen minutes and rub the nipples a little to stimulate them. Not only will the other person find this excruciatingly uncomfortable, but it's good for them too.

CHAPTER SIX

# *Erotic Pain*

## HOW CAN ANYTHING THAT HURTS BE GOOD?

*About three years ago, my husband read your book and ever since then he has been telling me that he wants me to whip him before we have sex. He says this excites him! Reading your book has perverted his mind. I have tried to get him to see a counselor but he refuses. He says he was always this way. He insists that there is nothing wrong with him or what he wants. I couldn't disagree more! His desires are unnatural. How can anything that causes pain be good for him or for us? Even though you try to make excuses for them, the practices you advocate are sick.*

Every so often I receive angry E-mail from people who believe that their partners have gone astray (or have been led astray) by exposure to a sex book, a piece of pornography, or an Internet site that features kinky sex. The rage they feel certainly presents a new set of challenges in the relationship. That is why the subject of kink should be discussed as carefully and thoughtfully as possible with a potentially hostile mate.

That said, the fact is that people cannot be led astray by exposure to pornography or discussions of kinky sex if something about those activities doesn't strike a chord with their existing sexuality. It's really just common sense. When people see something that truly doesn't interest them, their usual response will be either a "ho-hum" or a "yuck," and they'll turn away from it. If they stop to gape in rapt fascination, then, um, obviously they're fascinated. No matter how many times I have watched a video or read about women having sex with each other, as a heterosexual they've never inspired in me any bisexual fantasies.

On the other hand, the first time I read an SM story, it inspired lots of fantasies.

When a person has a powerful reaction to an unusual type of sexuality, it may be because what they are seeing stirs an intense emotional longing for the act, a desire often so hidden the person him- or herself may not be aware that it is there or may not have been aware until that moment. So it is possible that a partner's interest in whipping may remain dormant or latent for many years until it is awakened by discovering that there are others like himself.

Sometimes a person may know she has unusual fantasies and feelings yet not realize that she fits into any descriptive clinical category, such as "fetishist" or "masochist." For most people, these labels are alienating because they are associated with mental illness. It can be quite a revelation when people discover that the fantasies they have secretly harbored all their lives, and which they never labeled one way or another, fit the clinical definitions of common perversions. Even if they always knew whipping turned them on, it may take years before they can accept that this need is not evil, and that it is possible to fulfill such fantasies in a loving relationship.

Sexual identity is formed very early in life—perhaps by the time we are three or four, according to some sexological theorists. Our sexual identities will respond to environment, and will be affected by positive and negative feedback throughout the course of our lives. So, for example, someone with bondage fantasies who repeatedly has terrible experiences with bondage may, over time, simply shut down that part of his fantasy life because he learns to associate it with unhappiness. And, conversely, someone with only a slight fetish may, over time, develop a much more intense fetish if he repeatedly has pleasurable, exciting experiences.

This evolution of sexual desires, however, should not be confused with the formation of our fundamental sexual identity in early childhood. The formation process creates the template of our sexual identities; later experiences refine and modify that template. Dr. John Money, an eminent theorist on paraphilia (the clinical term for perversion), identifies the process as "lovemapping," in which each individual is born with a basic genetic predisposition that is progressively modified by experience and environment over the course of a lifetime.

If your partner needs pain in his or her erotic life, reading about others who feel the same will, at most, give him the courage and conviction to pursue his needs. It will not fundamentally change the person you've always known. He or she was always kinky, even if he didn't tell you or ask you to satisfy his urges.

Now, to address some common misperceptions about the pain itself. Pleasure in pain is not unnatural for human beings, although it may seem paradoxical. We are taught, from childhood on, to fear and loathe pain. Indeed, some people in our culture are raised with so morbid a fear of pain that they fear pain more than they fear death. However, the willing experimentation with pain is documented throughout human history. You needn't pore over books. Observe young children and you will note that among the pleasurable things they do to themselves, they also freely experiment with things we know to be painful, such as picking at scabs, cutting themselves, sticking sharp things into their orifices, butting their heads against walls or other children, and acting out other games that make adults stutter and gasp—and occasionally rush them to emergency rooms.

Although most parents will train their children out of doing things that hurt or can be harmful, some children learn from their early experiments that they actually enjoy rough play. They do not interpret the pain as a bad thing, even if they do feel it as pain. Behaviorally, they may have been in circumstances early in their lives where they associate pain with something positive. One example would be young children who undergo extensive, unpleasant medical treatments. They may cope with the pain by learning to associate it with attention and affection from adults. Others may cope by turning it into a game or accepting that the pain is necessary "for their own good." Ultimately, some percentage of these individuals grow up with an adult appetite for reenacting these scenarios.

A non-erotic example of the willing acceptance of pain would be rough contact sports. Is it truly necessary, say, for hockey players to beat each other with their sticks? Do football plays always justify the kind of violence we see on the field? (It goes without saying that boxing, wrestling, and Roller Derby are essentially about pain.) Most athletes willingly endure pain, and indeed may seem to take a perverse delight in giving and receiving pain on the field. Much of it, undoubtedly, is the positive feedback loop: It is considered heroic for athletes to subject their own bodies to intense physical hardship and to batter their opponents. They are rewarded for the spectacle of pain with money, social prestige, and praise.

Ballerinas too are famous masochists: The agony that classical dancers endure to perfect their technique is something they silently accept for the sake of their art, and something balletomanes expect of them.

So if we look at pain as an ordinary part of life, which people gladly endure for a variety of reasons, rather than as something uniquely sexual, it's easy to see that pain is not unnatural. It is, in fact, appropriate to certain professions, certain situations, and certain personalities.

Now, we don't yet know why some people get an erotic thrill from pain. There is considerable speculation (so far unsupported by data) that extreme sexual masochists may be genetically predisposed to interpret painful stimuli as pleasurable ones. According to this theory, a masochist's DNA, brain chemicals, and nervous system may show slight differences from the norm. If brain chemicals do determine masochism, people may well turn out to be engineered by God or nature to find pain sexy.

The bottom line: The problem isn't that one's partner is aroused by pain. The problem is that the couple cannot agree about what constitutes a satisfying or moral sex life.


## GOOD PAIN VS. BAD PAIN

*My lover and I have been doing D&S for the past year. Until now, it's mostly been bondage, and more sensual things like psychological dominance and control. Lately, I've been using light whips on her breasts and her buttocks to amazing effect. Her orgasms have been twice as intense. I believe she could go much fur-*

*ther with this, and she agrees. She says that she would like to take more pain, because that would make her feel more "owned" by me. Still, she is a little nervous about it, and I am hesitating because I want to make sure that I don't overstep her limits and end up giving her more than she can take. Do you have any advice for us on how to improve her tolerance to pain? Is it better to give someone one kind of pain than another kind?*

There is no question that there are two kinds of pain for a kinky bottom or submissive: First there is good pain and then there is bad pain.

Actually, it's helpful to think of "good pain" as "intense stimulation," because pain carries so many negative connotations. When a person experiences pain as a good feeling, or at least as a desirable feeling, it crosses the mysterious border between discomfort and delight and becomes a positive experience. Although there are general patterns we can identify, each person who enjoys pain puts just a slightly different spin on it, and gets something just slightly different out of it.

"Good pain" is so subjective and personal an experience that even the most articulate submissives find it difficult to explain. In conversations with hundreds of people over the years about *why* it is they enjoy pain, or what makes a particular kind of pain feel good when another type of pain (such as having dental work done, or stubbing a toe) feels so awful, most simply can't find the language to describe the emotional experience. They can describe the mechanics ("I love the thud" or "The precise burning pain of a cane really sinks into me") but not why a sensation they recognize as painful is so sexy to them. (Which is why so many people, when asked why they like something kinky, will only say, "Because it's fun!")

As I said, there are some general categories most people fall into, even if they don't entirely define their experience. For example, those who are interested in power dynamics say that pain has a meaning well beyond the sheer physical stimulus. The pain represents the power that the dominant has over the submissive. This could be the power simply to torment the submissive whenever the dom wishes or the authority to use pain for punishment (with the underlying assumption that the dominant has the right to punish the submissive for misbehavior). Pain represents the reality of the power relationship, and it is that reality of the power which the submissive finds exhilarating.

Some submissives genuinely dislike pain. One of my closest submissive friends says that pain scares him, and that he hates the discomfort. Yet he can't stop fantasizing about pain scenarios because to him a woman who has the power to hurt him, who enjoys hurting him, and who will hurt him despite his fears and anxiety, is the epitome of erotic dominance. His masochism is more psychological than physical, yet the physical pain satisfies his psychological cravings.

There are those who would not exactly qualify either as submissives or as masochists yet who have, in a sense, made a fetish of particular types of pain. Unlike SMers and masochists who may experiment with nearly any kind of painful stimulation, people who identify as "spankers" (and "spankees") often limit their kink entirely to pain to the buttocks and prefer only implements associated with spankings.

Spankers are seldom interested in the spectrum of intense stimuli or in the toys associated with SM (such as whips and floggers). Instead, the ritual of spanking and the action of slapping a bottom is the extent of their interest and experimentation with intense stimulus. Spankings are associated with pleasure in their minds, while other types of pain seem merely unpleasant.

Spankers are the most distinct group within the kinky communities to have this firm limit around the type of pain-play they will do, but the range of variation among individuals is extremely broad. There are, for example, many masochistic men who crave pain to their genitals but have no interest in receiving pain to any other part of their anatomy. I knew a man once, for example, who had a lifelong fascination with having his testicles crushed. His fantasies revolved around the idea of an attractive young woman kicking him in his groin. No other type of pain entered these fantasies and he did not identify as a masochist or a sadomasochist, because he associated those labels with whippings and spankings, activities that held no appeal to him whatsoever.

Similarly, it is fairly common for people whose kinkiness is focused on particular types of role-play to pursue only pain that would be appropriate to those scenarios. One example would be people who are excited by creating hospital or medical fantasies with their lovers. A "cruel nurse" or "evil doctor" might inflict pain on a partner using catheters or needles, but paddles and canes are unlikely to make an appearance in their erotic hospital room. The conventional SM toys simply don't fit with these scenarios.

In pony-play, where one partner is treated as a pony or a horse, it would be appropriate to use equestrian equipment, including crops, whips, bats, and other painful toys. But, again, you are unlikely to see a paddle or a cane, or medical equipment or nipple clamps, anywhere in sight. Those toys are (dare I say it?) for a horse of another color.

There are also individuals whose interest in pain is distinctly fetishistic, such as foot fetishists who are aroused by delivering pain only to feet. They may put their submissive partners into supremely tight shoes, or shoes whose heels are so high they force the foot into an excruciatingly unnatural position. In its own way, the pain is as cruel as any other, yet the only device used is a shoe.

Ticklers are another group who focus on a particular type of torment. They will tickle feet or underarms, bringing their partners to paroxysms of hysterical agony without ever picking up a whip or positioning a clamp. A majority of ticklers, indeed, do not consider themselves sadomasochists (or D&Sers) because they do not use any SM toys or have an explicit power dynamic with their partners.

Perhaps the most important aspect of good versus bad pain is context. Context is what explains why an unexpected, unwanted type of pain (such as bumping into a wall) is just as likely to be disagreeable to a masochist as it is to anyone else. For some people, in order for the context to be "right," there must be a conscious force behind the pain—a dominant or a top who delivers or inflicts the pain. For a D&Ser, the power dynamic is at the heart of the pain-play, and pain that occurs in any other context is just garden-variety awfulness.

Finally, it is well known that the greater a person's arousal, the higher his or her threshold (and desire) for intense stimulation. Just as people enjoy rougher caresses, harder thrusting, pinching, biting, or other sensations as their intercourse grows increasingly passionate, a masochist's or bottom's hunger for sensation also increases with arousal. Pain turns them on and, once they are turned on, the capacity and the need for pain grows in a gradually accelerating cycle.

In some individuals, this cycle or feedback loop between pain and sexual excitement is so overwhelming that they can climax from the pain alone, without direct manipulation of their sex organs. Men and women alike have been known to achieve orgasm from spankings and whippings.

Here, then, is a simple chart to explain the differences between the good and the bad.

| Good Pain | Bad Pain |
|---|---|
| a. is willingly received | a. is unwanted |
| b. intensifies arousal | b. dampens arousal |
| c. brings satisfaction | c. creates unhappiness |
| d. fits into an erotic context | d. has no erotic context |
| e. can lead to ecstasy | e. never stops feeling bad |

## HOW TO TAKE YOUR LOVER FROM PAIN TO PLEASURE: FIVE TIPS

If your partner has requested or consented to exploring painful stimuli as part of your erotic repertoire together, here are five techniques you can use to gently push the envelope, listed according to level of expertise. If you are completely new to this, start at technique one and perfect it before you move on to technique two. You may never go all the way to technique five, and that is perfectly fine.

Remember that before you do pain-play, you must:
• Talk to your partner carefully about what you have in mind.
• Establish clearly that you are mutually interested in trying this.
• Obtain your partner's explicit consent.

As I stress throughout the book, a clear understanding of your partner's limits, and an absolute respect for those limits, is a nonnegotiable element of consensual kink.

At the end of the chapter, I discuss some vital safety issues in more detail, but the main thing to keep in mind is that your interactions should be "safe, sane, consensual."

## 1. Start Small

If you have not previously experimented much with pain, do not go out right now and purchase a cabinet full of whips and paddles. Instead, use the standard equipment that has served sadomasochists for millennia: your hands. Have your partner get into a relaxed position, perhaps lying comfortably on a bed, and preferably nude. Slowly explore different areas of your partner's body with your fingertips. Press, prod, poke, and pinch flesh gently, watching your partner's reactions. Is he or she excited or fearful or a little of both? Is he or she groaning or grunting, or getting hard, or growing wet? Or does your partner look pissed off? (Whoops! A bad sign!)

If you aren't sure whether the noises you are hearing or the body changes you're witnessing are the result of good pain or bad pain, *ask*. In plain English. You needn't be solicitous if that would ruin your cruel fantasy. A simple, snarling "How much does that hurt, slut?" or "Does that excite you, you naughty thing?" fits nicely into almost any evil scenario.

Use your first exploration into intense stimulation mainly to find out which parts of your lover's body are most sensitive. Make a study of your partner's hot spots and learn how to read his or her body language (squirming, flinching, sweating, flushing) and sounds (moans, gasps, whimpers, gurgles). Believe it or not, each of those things means something, so develop a sense of which weird sounds and movements indicate pleasure and which indicate discomfort. Those responses will guide you and help you learn how to elicit the exact reactions you want.

Some bottoms, by the way, will get frisky during pain-play. When you inquire if something hurts, they may shrug mischievously and say something snotty ("Oh, please, you couldn't hurt a fly!"). My, my, they can get uppity, those greedy masochists! So, in case you didn't realize it, such responses are a not-so-subtle way that subs may let you know that you can (and indeed *should*) pinch them a little harder.

Don't get mad. Get even.

## 2. Experiment with Different Types of Touch and Squeeze

Stick with your hands for now, but experiment with a much wider variety of sensations: pinch skin (and genitals), squeeze flesh hard in your hand, flick your partner's genitals with your fingernails, slap his or her buttocks and thighs, scrape your nails over sensitive areas (you know which areas are sensitive by now, right?). Use your teeth for love bites or hard sucking in places that make your partner squirm.

Move from area to area, resting only a couple of minutes in any given place, and devote special attention to the most sensitive areas. Aim to confuse and excite your partner with as wide a range of uncomfortable caresses as possible and see if you can bring your partner to a state of arousal simply with these rough and punishing touches. If your partner is obviously getting very turned on by what you are doing, do it harder.

You may find you never need to move on to toys. Or you may discover that you and your partner derive so much pleasure from pain-play that you are both eager to explore other possibilities.

## 3. Incorporate Bondage

Some people find it difficult to lay still during pain-play, and others simply find it more erotic to receive intense stimulation while bound. If you've already advanced beyond the first two steps in your erotic expeditions, try tying your partner up and running through technique two all over again. You may see more intense responses now, because the vulnerability of the bondage is likely to sharpen your partner's focus on every little thing you do.

## 4. Tease and Tempt Your Partner with Toys

If you are ready to use toys, or already own toys and want to delve deeper into pain scenarios, first learn to use the toys in a sensual manner to see if your partner can eroticize the toys themselves. If so, it will greatly enhance their receptivity to pain.

For example, take a whip from your collection and see how many different ways you can use it sensually on your partner before inflicting any painful sensations with it. No matter how harsh the implement, it's a good thing to know how to control it as a sensual toy before using it as a painful one. If you cannot bring your partner to at least an early stage of sexual arousal through sensual games with the toy, try another toy or keep practicing your techniques.

Run the handle over your partner's body, as if it was a penis or a dildo (or use the handle as a dildo); lightly run it over your partner's lips and command him or her to kiss it or suck it; let the lashes fall as gently as possible across their belly, back, breasts, thighs, and other sensitive areas. Swirl the lashes around softly, pulling them up between your partner's legs or drawing the tips softly over your partner's face.

As you work, the toy should gradually begin to feel like an extension of your own hand and fingertips. At the same time, your partner's erotic anticipation should build, intensifying his or her craving for more sensation. If you are a real genius at this, your partner will become so hungry for more sensation, he or she will beg you to use it harder or more cruelly. This is a very good thing!

Another excellent way to tease and tempt your partner into wanting more pain is to stop periodically during its harsh use and to revert back to sensual teasing. Letting your partner have a complete range of sensual/erotic experiences (and, in essence, a relationship) with the toy you are using will help him or her develop an instinctively erotic response to the toy each time you bring it out.

## 5. Advanced Pain

If you are long past the experimental phase and are seriously looking to expand a masochist's pain limits, it is time to get very serious about the equipment you use and to consider investing in a range of implements that can deliver a wide variety of sensations.

If whipping is your thing, you should try to have several different types of whips in your collection, beginning with a very light and sensual flogger whose main purpose is to warm up the skin. A whip with wide deerskin lashes is perfect for this. Learn which implements are harshest by giving your partner one hard, well-placed stroke with each (well placed means you deliver the pain to the buttocks or another area where you cannot cause damage).

Some advanced players develop a set routine in their painplay. For whippings, they begin with a selected lightweight flogger and move up the whipping food chain, finishing with something heavy and nasty. This is good as far as it goes. It stops short of spontaneity. On the other hand, if you enjoy ritual, this could be just the right approach for you.

When it comes to selecting your toys, there is no empirical hierarchy of pain. Different people respond differently to different implements. One person may find a paddle to be deliciously intense and another person may find it agonizingly unpleasant. I have known masochists who enjoyed an enormous amount of pain from a cane, yet who reached their limit almost immediately when a neuro-wheel (a medical device, reminiscent of a pizza cutter, which pricks the skin to test neurological response) is introduced. Objectively, the neuro-wheel is not meaner than a cane, but some people find the sharp, prickly sensation to be unendurable.

So it is up to you to discover what your partner can and cannot tolerate, and which particular implements trigger the kinds of reactions you want.

I recommend a wide range of toys for these explorations because it is helpful, in expanding limits, to keep changing sensations. The distraction alone of different types of pain, delivered at different intervals or for different amounts of time, helps continuously shift the submissive's or bottom's focus, and may assist him or her in accepting more pain. It also virtually eliminates the possibility of boredom, which is the antithesis of eroticism. I have known masochists who grew bored when tops just continually repeated the same spanking or whipping over and over and over again. There is just no excuse for boring your submissive.

So if you use a flogger (which delivers a pounding thud to a large area), then try a cat o' nine tails for a while (which delivers stinging pain over a large area), then switch to a small paddle (which delivers a sharp but thudding pain to a very small area), then pick up a crop (which delivers a sharp sting to a tiny area), and then return to the flogger, the submissive's concentration will continually shift. You will be able to take him or her on a kind of a voyage through pain, guiding them through peaks and valleys as their reactions to the different implements varies from "Ouch, that hurts!" to "Ouch, I love it!"

If you can take your partner on this voyage, you will be able continuously to expand their capacity for intense sensation. They will learn to adapt to what you want to give them, with little or no time to fixate on fears that may limit their ability to take the pain. Their sexual energy will be fully devoted to dealing with what you are doing. Nurturing their ability to follow your lead, and thus to surrender control over their responses to you, is the key to expanding their limits.

As a final note: No matter what your level of experience, I strongly recommend that you intersperse your pain-play with affectionate kisses and reassurance. Encouraging your partner through positive feedback ("You are such a good girl/boy to take this for me" or "I'm proud of how much pain you are taking") can make a real difference in your partner's attitude.

If mixing affection with SM is unattractive to you, then I recommend you at least end the pain-play with a nice, long hug. Holding your partner for a few minutes and saying something tender is even better. Positive reinforcement, and reassurance that you care about the person and approve of them, will help them to feel comfortable about their need for pain. Without the top's or dominant's emotional support, and clear signals that you truly appreciate their willing participation, some submissives may feel guilty or ashamed about enjoying pain or, worse, may feel abandoned or rejected by you.

## CAN I BE SUBMISSIVE IF I DON'T LIKE PAIN?

*I've been exploring the world of D&S for the past year. I know I am submissive because when I see pictures of other women in bondage or wearing a collar and leash I get so envious and turned on. I wish I was in their place. But I'm afraid to look for a master because I talked to some other submissives on AOL and they told me that it isn't enough to like bondage, I have to like pain too. I had bad experiences as a child and I don't want anyone to hit me, not even my master. My friends said that if I don't enjoy whippings and spankings I can't really serve someone. Now I'm confused. Can I still be someone's slave even if I don't like pain? Will any masters be interested in a "pain wimp" like me?*

One of the common misconceptions about BDSM and D&S is that it always involves pain-play. This is simply not true. Pain is for those who enjoy it. It is not the hallmark of all kinky relationships by any means.

If you are afraid of pain, have bad associations with being hit or otherwise hurt, or have zero tolerance for intense physical stimulation, it doesn't mean that you are any less submissive than someone who is physically masochistic.

What makes someone submissive, quite simply, is the desire to serve and obey. If you also desire to be owned by someone, then you might make someone a good slave. No matter what clueless people may tell you, there is no law that says you must endure things you don't like, and no biological model for the "ideal" submissive. Submissives are individuals, not clones. No one should put themselves under pressure to do things that turn them off. Where's the fun in that?

The particular types of kinky things you do with your partner should be shaped by who you are and what you need as a unique and precious human being. Indeed, there are just as many masochists who don't enjoy psychological submission as there are submissives who don't enjoy pain.

D&S relationships that do not involve pain-play are called "psychological" or "sensual" dominance. These terms imply that the relationship is based on verbal or mental control, without a pain component. The dominant gives the orders, makes the decisions, and controls the submissive's behavior in bed (and sometimes outside of it too). Instead of painful punishments, a "sensual dominant" chooses other paths, such as scoldings, restrictions of privileges, or assigning unpleasant or tedious tasks (anything from scrubbing floors and fixtures to writing something out hundreds of times).

When you search for a master, find out right up front if you and he are compatible on the issue of pain. Just as there are subs who don't want pain, there are dominants who don't want to inflict it. If you meet a man who must give pain to feel sexually alive, then he will not be a good match for you. Instead, seek out someone who appreciates what you have to offer in terms of submitting to bondage, serving his sexual needs, obeying him, and whatever other more sensual types of submission you fantasize about.

## SAFETY, SAFETY, SAFETY AND, IN CASE YOU WEREN'T LISTENING, SAFETY!

Here is a very short list of the most basic "do's" and "don'ts" of pain-play.

### Pain-Play Nevers

If you're the one receiving the pain:
  • Never drink alcohol or do drugs before pain-play. Intoxicants alter your perceptions of sensation and dull your capacity to judge whether the pain you're taking is enough or way

too much. If you can't take pain without getting high, then do not do it.

• Never agree to let someone you don't know use an intense piece of equipment on you.

• Never start any kind of pain-play without first discussing what you will be doing and establishing a clear way (such a safe word) to let the dominant know when you've reached a limit.

• Never assume that someone who owns a piece of equipment necessarily knows how to use it safely. If possible, watch the person use the equipment on someone else first, or check the person's reputation with people who know him or her. At the first sign that the person is clumsy or uninformed about basic health issues, use your safe word and stop the play. For example, if someone uses any implement to strike you on the lower back (near the kidneys), hits you in a bony area of your body (knees, ankles, on the spine, etc.), or keeps missing the target you've agreed on (such as buttocks), *stop the play.* Remember that you are a kinky sex partner, not a sacrificial lamb.

• Never conceal health or psychological issues of any kind. Do you have abuse issues or memories that could be triggered by a pain scenario? Would any particular type of pain-play exacerbate an existing medical condition? (For example, sharps and hemophilia don't mix; neither do latex allergies and rubber whips, hemorrhoids and large butt plugs, and so on.)

Before you begin any type of pain-play, tell the top about any challenges you may have, and make sure he or she not only understands your limits but will respect them unquestioningly.

• Never get so carried away by the experience that you lose all sense of what's going on with your own body. Pain-play stimulates endorphins and can put submissives into an ecstatic trance. Do your best to keep your wits about you so that you can use your safe word when appropriate.

If you're the one giving the pain:

• Never drink alcohol or do drugs before you give someone pain. Nothing hurts a dominant's judgment more than intoxicants. They make you unsteady, less mentally aware, and less emotionally caring. If you can't do SM without getting high first, then don't give pain.

• Never use equipment before learning how to use it safely. Most dominants will, at a minimum, test a new piece of equipment on themselves, usually by rapping or whipping a striking implement on their forearm to get a sense of its intensity. For any kind of extreme pain, or any advanced piece of equipment, your best bet is to attend a seminar offered at SM outreach or educational programs that will teach you the basic techniques you need to enact your fantasies sanely and safely.

Only idiots pick up a pain toy for the first time and start using it at full force. If you are too much of a coward to try it on yourself, you shouldn't be handling it in the first place. If you can't get to a seminar or find a book or magazine with detailed instructions on how to use a tool, then stick to sensual teasing (refer to "Start Small," page 130) until you master the implement and your technique.

• Never push someone to accept pain that they haven't explicitly agreed (consented) to take, and stop as soon as your partner uses his or her safe word or otherwise communicates that he or she has reached a limit. It is your responsibility to ensure that the pain-play remains a safe, pleasurable experience for your partner. Monitor your partners' reactions and ask them periodically how they are doing.

• Never use unclean equipment. All toys should be thoroughly cleaned the first time you use them, and after every use as well. It's the things you can't see—germs, bacteria, viruses—that pose the greatest threat to your partner's health. They may be present on metal, leather, and wood objects, and on any toy that strikes or enters the body.

• Never be lulled into a false sense of security by giving your partner a safe word. Pain-play can induce a kind of erotic trance in your partner, which impairs his or her ability to decide when to use a safe word. If your partner hyperventilates, becomes hysterical, or otherwise shows signs of extreme emotional distress, stop immediately and calm him or her down until you can determine whether it is safe to continue.

## TOP TORTURE TOYS AND TECHNIQUES

Here is a list of common ways to deliver intense sensation to your lover. I've divided the toys and techniques into two categories: Store-Bought Suffering (equipment that can be purchased at adult sex shops) and House and Garden Pain (techniques and things you can find around the house or yard).

Note: All toys may be used so gently as to produce only the mildest sensation. There is no law that says you have to use them for pain only—indeed, you'll see that some of the toys on the list are most frequently used for drama. But to help you understand more about them, I list guidelines on what kind of sensation they produce when used at full force.

### Store-Bought Suffering

*Whips:* May also be called flails, floggers, and cat o' nines. The single most available type of kinky toy, whips come in all sizes, materials, and designs. Most common are leather whips: The lashes are leather laces or strips and the handles are braided leather, sometimes around a solid (wood) core. Leather whips are medium to heavyweight. You can also find them with lashes made of rubber (intense), plastic (light to intense, depending on the plastic), silk/satin (very light), nylon (light to moderate), and horsehair (moderate). Some lashes are beaded or weighted at their ends (intense to very intense).

Bullwhips (very intense) are frequently seen but seldom used for striking. The reason is that it is very difficult to control a six-foot or longer whip, and all too easy to hit someone in the wrong spot. Most players use bullwhips for drama, by sporting one to intimidate people or by snapping it during a session to startle their partner with the frightening whistle and crack it makes. However, there are those who have mastered the bullwhip and whose ability to deliver a sharp, precise sting with it approaches an art form.

The single-tail whip resembles a short, stubby bullwhip. It has one sinewy, sensuous, yet ferocious braided lash (intense to very intense). Single-tail whips have developed a minor cult following as their unique combination of snakelike sensuality and pure viciousness delights many pain-players.

*Crops:* Available widely at adult sex shops (but much cheaper at tack shops), these consist of a stiff rod with a short, biting leather strip at the end (moderate). The cheap kind typically found at sex shops are often made of plastic; tack shops, which cater to upscale equestrians, carry finer, imported English models in leather.

Similar in design to crops are "bats" (also known as "county bats"), another piece of English equestrian equipment (moderate to intense). A bat is shorter than a crop, has a thicker rod, and the leather strip at the end is wider and usually thicker than a crop's.

*Paddles:* These come in a very wide variety of styles, sizes, and materials. The paddle purist usually prefers wooden types (moderate to very intense), either resembling something used for a fraternity hazing or similar to paddles used for school discipline. Wood paddles are typically rectangular, with narrowed handles that make them easier to hold. They may be made of lightweight wood (such as the wood used for Ping-Pong paddles) or heavy woods (such as oak). Some paddles have holes drilled in them to reduce air resistance (intense to very intense). The airflow through the holes helps to produce a more vicious wallop.

Leather paddles are also fairly common. The paddle may be made of a single thick piece of leather or of two thick pieces glued together (moderate); some are reinforced by steel or another metal bolster beneath the leather (intense to very intense).

Also known as a "split paddle," a tawse is a wide leather strap split into strips at the end (light to intense). A design variation on the tawse is a "devil's hand" (moderate to intense), which is a leather paddle cut to resemble a three-fingered hand. A devil's hand is usually made of reinforced leather (or two thick pieces of leather sewn or glued together).

Although not technically a paddle, wood hairbrushes (moderate to intense) also are favored by many spankers and may occasionally be found in sex shops (though it's cheaper to pick one up at a supermarket). Spanking is done with the smooth side. Some people also use the brush side, scraping it across the skin to increase sensitivity during a spanking.

*Rods and Canes:* Spare the rod and spoil the sadomasochist?

The kind of rod (intense to very intense) you may find in an adult toy store is more likely to be made of plastic or fiberglass than the old-fashioned type made of wood, but the principle is the same and the sensations range from moderate to very intense. Most rods have a handle whose materials vary but tend towards synthetics.

Like rods, canes are sticklike implements (intense to very intense). The natural type are made of bamboo or rattan (see under "Nature's Toys" in "House and Garden Pain," page 145). The wood is dressed and sometimes finished by wrapping leather around one end to protect the palm of the person doing the caning. They may also have a curved handle, like an orthopedic cane. Canes for hitting people are made of the reedy shoots of plants. They are thin, extremely lightweight, and very flexible. They should not be confused with the canes that are used as walking sticks; these are made of hardwoods, are heavyweight and inflexible, and are therefore unsafe to use on anyone.

*Neuro-Wheel:* A stainless-steel medical device used by doctors to check neurological responses, this is a spiked wheel set into a slender, ribbed handle (intense to very intense). It looks like a cross between a spur and an old-fashioned pizza cutter and can be used to prick or even lightly pierce the skin, depending on how hard it's pressed into the skin. Available in many BDSM shops but cheaper through medical- and scientific-supply catalogues. (See "Sharps," page 144.)

*Painful/Restrictive Bondage Devices:* A range of bondage toys may be used to deliver pain, including clips, clamps, clothespins, butterfly boards, and much more. Indeed, most restraints and bondage toys will cause discomfort or pain if the bottom is left bound for long periods of time or placed in awkward positions.

For a complete discussion of bondage devices, refer to chapter 5 on erotic bondage. The only thing I will mention in depth here is the corset.

At its most restrictive, a corset with boning or other reinforcement can produce intense pain. Even when the corset is not very tightly laced, it still produces a certain amount of distress to the body. By compressing the torso, a corset places stress not only on the flesh but on the underlying organs and the skeleton (particularly the pelvis and ribs).

Cross-dressers and female fans of ladies' lingerie generally endure the discomforts of corsetting to improve their appearance and not because they actually enjoy the pain. "Corset masochists," however, may enjoy the way their bodies look as a result of corsetting but are specifically interested in the pain and restrictiveness of the garment.

Boned corsets are available primarily at fetish fashions boutiques and high-quality lingerie shops.

*Electrotorture Devices:* These are adult toys that generate a low-level electrical charge (moderate to very intense). The most readily available one is the "violet wand," an old quack medical device used to stimulate muscle tissue. It consists of a hard-bodied casing you hold in your hand. On one end is a wire that runs to a static-electricity generator with control knobs to adjust intensity. On the opposite end, glass attachments of various sizes and shapes (included with the kit) are inserted. When the attachment is placed close to skin, the glass glows purple and a static shock is discharged.

A handful of BDSM merchants specialize in electro-toys.

*Anal Toys:* Adult toys designed to fit into the rectum are *not* manufactured for pain-play but for pleasurable anal penetration. They may enhance a bottom's arousal by causing him or her to feel plugged or full; submissives, meanwhile, may be aroused by the humiliation of having their anuses controlled this way.

That said, I include anal toys here because some models can cause discomfort, particularly to someone who is unused to anal-play. If used with deliberate sadism, or misused, they can cause extreme discomfort (intense to very intense).

Among the toys available for anal penetration are anal plugs (also known as butt plugs), dildos, anal beads, and horsehair tails with insertable handles (used in pony-play). The discomfort level, when used properly on a relaxed partner, is zero to moderate. Lubrication further reduces discomfort.

The chief difference between a butt plug and a dildo is that a butt plug has a flared base to prevent it from going too deeply into the rectum. Either type may look like a real penis, veins and all, and be made of flexible rubber; or they may be made of hard plastic and have an elongated, phallic (but not realistically penile) shape. It's commonly accepted that a dildo is something that's moved around (in and out) while a plug is generally left in place for a period of time.

Anal beads (also known as a "string of pearls") consist of a series of wooden beads or rubber balls strung on a leather cord. Anal beads range in size from small to large. If you've ever seen stuff in sex shops that look like big rubber oranges on a string and wondered what they were, well, now you know. Anal beads are inserted during sex. When the bottom reaches climax, his or her partner slowly tugs on the exposed end. The balls pop out, one by one, stimulating the anus (moderate to very intense). Needless to say, the bigger the bead or ball, the more intense the stimulation.

Anal toys are sometimes used to stretch out a bottom's anus so that he or she can more easily accommodate anal intercourse or anal fisting—or, with a submissive or slave, for the erotic humiliation and helplessness this invasive form of play induces.

One may also occasionally see an inflatable butt plug. This is a hollow rubber dildo with an attached air pump that inflates the plug to the desired size, again to stretch the rectum. (Obviously for those who are turned on by stretching, this won't be painful but will enhance their anal pleasure.)

## House and Garden Pain

*Unguents/Irritants/Abrasives:* A look into one's pantry, kitchen cabinets, and tool chest will yield some of the common products that sadomasochists incorporate into their pain-play. These include Ben-Gay, mineral ice, hot sauce, chili peppers, and peppermint extract, all of which cause a stinging or burning sensation. Typical abrasives are pumice, sandpaper, and steel wool, and they produce a scratching, scraping, or burning sensation.

Any of the above may be rubbed into or against skin, whether it's the buttocks or the genitals (light to very intense).

*Fire and Ice:* Hot wax (discussed in the bondage chapter) has become a very popular form of pain-play. At its lightest, it is only sensual, with the wax dripped from enough of a distance that it only feels warm on the skin. However, intense players will bring the candle closer so that the hot wax causes a strong burning sensation (or even a minor burn). A candle used for hot wax should not contain artificial dyes. They have higher melting temperatures and can cause burns.

Ice cubes (also discussed in the bondage chapter) are an interesting alternative, especially when used to cool down skin that has been tormented. Some kinksters play with "ice dildos." They fill condoms with water and freeze them, then rub the dildos over their partners' bodies or insert them into their body cavities. Depending on your partner's body sensitivity, ice produces sensations anywhere from light to intense.

*Sharps:* Sharps include any metal implement with an extremely sharp tip or a blade. Sterile needles, sterile syringes, knives, and razors are the most popular items to fall into this category. Needless to say (or is that "needles to say"?), you can expect all sharps to cause intense to very intense pain.

The absolute equipment safety standard here is sterility. Because sharps may draw or otherwise come in contact with blood, they can transmit the AIDS virus, hepatitis, and other diseases when shared. Unclean sharps, even when used only on one person, may carry germs and cause serious infections. It is therefore critical that anyone who plays with sharps knows exactly how to sterilize them (according to medical standards) before or after each use.

Sterile needles are used for "play-piercing" or "temporary

piercing": This is when the needle is inserted through a nipple, scrotal sac, labia, or other area of skin.

As gruesome as it may sound, needle-play is a fairly noninvasive and moderate-risk activity. The holes are minute and the sensation is more like pricking than stabbing. Sterile syringes may be used in the same way, to the same effect.

Knives and razors are most often shown or waved about to heighten the sense of danger and the atmosphere of fear. However, some people use sharps on their partner. Knives are most popular in conjunction with bondage; tops may cut off the bottom's clothes with knives, slipping the blunt edge of the knife under the ropes or clothes and against the bottom's skin, then pulling the knife up towards them, shredding as they go. (Never ever place the blade down against the skin when cutting someone out of ropes or clothes.)

A small percentage of pain-players use knives and razors for pain, and will use the tips to prick skin or hold the blade against the skin, lightly abrading the flesh, scraping off hair or inflicting superficial cuts. (Scalpels and straight razors may also be used in this way.)

When sharps cut or pierce skin and draw blood, the practice is called "blood sports." Blood sports and sharp-play frightens a lot of people because if the person doesn't know what he or she is doing, serious injury could result. The high-risk nature of these types of pain-play make them controversial in the Scene and the subject of aggressive debate.

*Nature's Toys:* A backyard, park, or wildlife area offers several natural alternatives that have become popular with sadomasochists. The most common plants that yield painful implements are bamboo, cane, nettles, and birch trees.

The stalks of bamboo and cane plants are, indeed, natural canes (moderate to very intense). The type that are commercially available are cleaned up and finished canes from these common plants.

Nettles are used to irritate and scratch skin. (The thorny stems of roses are sometimes used as well.) The abrading sensation ranges from moderate to intense.

Smallish, slender branches from birch trees may be bundled and used as a natural whip. SMers aren't the only ones to enjoy the light to intense sensations of being beaten by birches: Birch whips have been used to stimulate and invigorate skin in saunas and steam rooms around the world for millennia.

# CHAPTER SEVEN

# Fetishism

## WHAT'S A FETISH?

*Two weeks ago, after having a few too many, my fiancé suddenly confessed that he "has a fetish." He passed out right afterwards, so I never found out what he meant. Since then, he's refused to discuss it with me! I wish I knew what he meant! Was he saying that he owns a fetish? Like, is he keeping a shrunken head or a dried-up rabbit's foot in a drawer somewhere? Or does he mean he has a fetish for something, like a shoe or something? He acts so ashamed whenever I bring it up I'm almost afraid he is hiding something gross from me. Do you think I should make him tell me before we get married?*

Lovers can be so romantic, can't they? Drunk one minute, unconscious the next.

The English word *fetish* can be traced back to the medieval Portuguese word *fetich,* which refers to religious relics believed to possess magical properties. Early Christians frequently attributed metaphysical powers to such things as the severed arms, fingers, skulls, and other bones of saints, or the garments saints once wore. People believed that the relics themselves could perform miracles through an invested spirit power from God. Many still do, as witness the Shroud of Turin.

When fifteenth-century Portuguese explorers arrived in West Africa and discovered that local peoples believed that their religious carvings possessed similar spirit powers, the word *fetich* was applied to their holy artifacts as well. Eventually, people came to associate the word *fetish* uniquely with the religious art of pagan (including Native American) societies, but, in fact, it is the product of a Christian worldview. Indeed, Roman Catholic churches still store sacred objects assumed to possess spiritual magic in reliquaries behind the altar.

In the nineteenth century, scientists exploring the brave new world of human sexuality co-opted "fetishism" to describe their patients' erotic fascinations for objects or body parts. To "have a fetish" now means to be extremely turned on by some thing or some aspect of someone's body (a foot, facial hair, a belly button, and so on). Most fetish objects are articles of dress or other items that come in close contact with the body.

The early sexologists demonstrated a remarkable sensitivity in associating "fetish" with an object of erotic fascination. As with a religious fetish, an erotic fetish too possesses magic powers: It has the power to arouse emotions and to inspire sexual ecstasy.

While the general perception of fetishes and fetishists seems to be that they are weird, in fact fetishism is a common phenomenon. Indeed, in its very broadest sense, fetishism is a normal aspect of the human psyche. We are all capable, and even likely, to believe that inanimate objects can change our fortunes.

Do you own a lucky marble or coin? Is there a good-luck medallion hanging around your neck? Do you pray to a statue or symbol? Is there a special piece of clothing you wear to bring you (or your team) good luck? Do you believe a crystal or a copper bracelet has healing properties? Whether you kiss the Blarney Stone, a cross, or a mezuzah, you are expressing the near-universal belief that things we know to be nonliving are, in fact, capable of performing divine miracles.

Collectors too are fetishists: They become intently focused on a category of objects (from jelly jars to seashells), and accumulate them largely for the pleasure of owning and admiring them. The things they acquire develop special meaning to them. Sometimes they are believed to bring good luck. They always have the power to make their owners inexplicably happy.

Clotheshorses are fetishists of a sort, and not only when they buy kinky clothes. Ask a woman who owns hundreds of pairs of shoes why exactly she needs them all, or why she bought those fur-trimmed, powder-blue satin mules that would stain if you breathed on them. There is no rational explanation. As with handbags, furs, scarves, and other luxury items, shoes possess powers above and beyond their functional use. Indeed, that is part of their mystique and appeal.

Even the leathery truck driver who stops at swap meets to pick up a few new matchbooks or beer cans for his collection back home may be said to be a fetishist. For whatever reason, the objects he collects have a value to him that cannot be explained by their real value, much less their practical use.

Unfortunately, fetishes that make people directly sexually aroused are separated out from the norm and viewed as tainted. In other words, if you collect hundreds of items mainly for the satisfaction of owning them, you are considered normal; if you collect hundreds of items because they give you a sexual thrill, you are considered sick. Personally, if I went to the trouble of collecting something, I'd want to get the biggest bang for my buck. A free sexual thrill seems like a good deal to me.

Be that as it may, some sexual fetishes are accepted in our culture. These are fetishes a majority of people seem to share, or at least which a majority feel fairly comfortable admitting that they share. Breasts are the most obvious example: North American culture is boob-o-centric. Entertainment media and medical science alike have allowed, and even encouraged, men and women to fixate on milk glands. The fascination with breasts may seem perfectly natural to us, but in cultures where other body parts are considered much sexier, our national breast fixation seems like a pretty strange fetish.

Scientific theories about sexual fetishes are incomplete at best. Some new and promising ones are based on current research into brain structure. The data suggests that there may be areas of the brain that control fetishistic impulses and that, therefore, are affected by brain chemicals.

Other theories are purely speculative, if not downright whimsical. Freudian and neo-Freudian analysts, for example, suggest that fetishism is a triggered response resulting from intense sexual shame. They've speculated that people develop fetishes because, in childhood, they accidentally saw a parent naked and, in grievous dread of seeing the sexual organs, looked away in shame (usually downward, to the feet) and were erotically imprinted for life. The sexual desire triggered by the glimpse of the genitals was permanently redirected to whatever the child gazed on next, as was the trauma and guilt.

Another theory holds that people develop fetishes because of similarly pivotal—but pleasant—experiences in early childhood. For example, a small child may crawl over to an adult's foot and in that moment may coincidentally be sexually excited. The child forever afterwards feels a sexual charge at the sight and smell of feet, because he learned to associate the feet with his accidental arousal.

Both theories are woefully half-baked. For one, if all it takes is crawling, coincidental excitement, or sexual shame at the sight of a parent's nakedness to cause fetishism, how many children would not be slated for kinkiness? Next, while these theories work for foot fetishes, they don't quite explain the thousands of other fetish objects that drive people mad with lust. Were they too, at one time or another, the next thing a child saw after looking away from his parent's genitals? I am trying to imagine under what circumstances a child would be likely to avoid staring at his mother's naked thighs and end up, instead, gazing at a jockstrap or rubber raincoat.

Another theory that's never been scientifically validated, and which is contradicted by anecdotal information, is that "true" fetishists are all men. Most contemporary studies have relied on male subjects, although case studies dating back to the nineteenth century have chronicled female fetishists. I believe that the reason we think of only men as fetishists is because of the ongoing Victorian bias in the psychiatric community that men are more sexually driven than women and therefore more likely to be sexually perverse. Because of this assumption, women may not be asked the kinds of questions about their sexuality that would yield reliable data on their fetishes.

Indeed, many women probably don't realize that their intense erotic fascinations with objects or devices (whether it's a fur, a blanket, shoes, or a sex toy) meet the clinical definition of fetishism. This may explain why men make up the larger part of the clinical drift (the people who drift into therapists' office). If you don't know something's a sexual problem, it's unlikely you'll be looking for counseling.

To my mind, the idea that a powerful sexual fixation must be male, or primarily male, is an expression of the outdated belief that women are not as highly sexed as men. It is without basis in reality. As a woman who has fetishes, and as a researcher who's interviewed numerous other female fetishists, I know that female fetishism is a very real and regular phenomenon.

I know one woman whose preferred way of achieving orgasm is to have a man she knows model high-heels shoes. The higher and pointier the heel, the more it excites her. She asks the man to walk back and forth while she masturbates. For the finale, she has him raise his foot to the bed, bringing the shoe within inches of her face as she climaxes.

I'd call that a true shoe fetish.

While sexual fetishes may be disquieting to someone who doesn't share them, they are usually harmless. As with all types of perversion, they cannot be cured. More than that, you cannot choose your fetish. No one wakes up one day and decides that he would rather be turned on by galoshes than by breasts. All one can say authoritatively is that they seem to be innate predilections that develop differently in different individuals.

What can cause problems in a relationship, however, is when the fetishist cannot have a complete sexual encounter without his fetish. While most fetishists can have satisfying sex without the fetish, or simply by privately fantasizing about it, there are some hard-core fetishists who cannot climax unless their fetish is close. An accommodating spouse can deal with this simply by including the fetish object in all intimate encounters. But not everyone can be that accommodating, particularly if they feel threatened by the fetish.

Some partners of fetishists develop insecurities or a sense of rivalry with the fetish objects. They worry that their partner cares more about the object, or is more excited by the object, than he or she is about the spouse. Some fetishists aggravate the problem by directing their erotic energy to the fetish object and paying little or no attention to their lover's needs.

As frustrating as this situation can be, the problem isn't the fetish; it's that your partner is behaving selfishly. Ignoring a partner's needs and thinking only of getting one's own jollies from sex is not exactly unique to fetishists. A bad lover is a bad lover and his or her bad behavior needs to be addressed.

If your partner lets his fetish get in the way of your mutual satisfaction, then you need to work together on improving his or her sensitivity in bed. You can, in fact, use the fetish as a bargaining chip. "I'll wear your favorite boots if you do X for me" is one bit of romantic bribery that might work. Let your partner know, in subtle ways or direct ones (depending on your personality), that sexual satisfaction is a two-way street and that if he or she expects you to go along with fetish-play, you expect equal pleasure in return. Use the communications tools in the early chapters of this book to help open an honest dialogue with your partner on how to improve your sex life as a team.

### A FETISH IS ALIVE!

*I was staying at my brother's place last week, sitting for his dog while he was out of town. One night, I was looking for a sweatshirt I could borrow to go walk the dog, and in one of his closets I found the most incredible assortment of ladies' shoes that I had ever seen. I always knew my brother was weird, but I couldn't figure out what he was doing with all those women's shoes. When he came home, I confronted him and asked him what that was about. He told me he was a shoe fetishist and assured me that he didn't wear them himself, he just liked to keep them around. At that point, we were both too embarrassed to say anything else. But there's something I still don't understand. What do fetishists do with their shoes? Does he just sit and look at them at night or is there more to this? Do I want to know?*

What looks like a simple shoe to you is something much more meaningful to a shoe fetishist: It has a living spirit. Fetishists make love to that spirit with their bodies, their souls, their words, and their minds. Since fetish objects are perceived as having a spirit all their own, in some respects a fetishist relates to them as if they were living things. In this way, although nonfetishists may find it mystifying, fetishists can have satisfying relationships with the object of their erotic fascination.

The relationship between fetishist and fetish is individual to each person. For some, the relationship is purely romantic and sexual. There are foot fetishists, for example, who find it profoundly satisfying, emotionally and erotically, to kiss and lick toes for hours. They find toes aesthetically appealing. They find them tasty. The toes are as sexy to them as nipples or lips might be to another person. Indeed, for some people the fetish object may be a substitute for a sex organ. Men may make love to it with their penises or women may use a fetish object as a dildo.

For others, the fetish may have a special symbolism. Another woman I knew had a fetish for leather belts—not just because of the leather smell, which turned her on, but also because the belt symbolized sadism to her, as she had many deep fantasies about being hit and whipped by belts. Kissing a belt may have been erotic to her, but the real power of the belt was its ritual significance as something that delivered a kind of pain that both aroused her and made her feel submissive. When she smelled the leather, or heard someone talk about a belt, her relationship with her fetish was instantly engaged. She got that delicious fluttering of arousal that someone else might get at the mention of kissing.

It's impossible, therefore, to know for a certainty what any particular fetishist does with his shoes unless he tells you. He could possibly get his greatest satisfaction from touching them, arranging them, and enjoying them on a purely sensual and aesthetic level. Or the shoes could have a symbolic meaning to him—for example, he might enjoy fantasizing about women wearing them and stepping on him in them. He might create the fantasy scenarios by himself to satisfy his kinky needs. Equally likely is that he enjoys making love to his shoes the way you might enjoy making love to your significant other.

## FETISH TALES

The most common question I get from fetishists is simply "Am I the only one?" This is the number one anxiety that fetishists feel: that no one could possibly understand their feelings, much less share them.

In my experience, no one is ever alone. No matter how unusual or bizarre the fetish, someone is likely to share it with you. The Internet has proved this to me again and again. I will stumble across a fetish that I have never heard discussed anywhere or seen catalogued in any scholarly text, and to my amazement will observe that as soon as one Web site exists for the fetish, others begin springing up, clearly demonstrating that the audience and need is there. It is usually just a matter of someone stepping forward and admitting to a particular fetish before others will suddenly appear, confessing to having the same one.

While doing some research on fetishes ten years ago, I came across someone who related an extended story about his fetish for toy balloons. His biggest fantasy was to have sex with a woman while she wore balloons. He wanted to tape balloons on her naked body and hear them pop as they made love. The sound of the popping would bring him to orgasm. In other words, when they popped, so did he. He had been searching, unsuccessfully, for a girlfriend who would indulge this fantasy on a regular basis. Thus far, he had convinced a couple of dates to try out his fetish but none of the relationships lasted longer than a few noisy dates.

His account of this fantastic fetish bemused me. I'd never heard of anything like it, or seen anything written about it before. It seemed so unlikely that I even wondered if the whole thing was just a fiction or a wacky prank.

Shoot ahead about eight years to the advent of the Web and the proliferation of fetish sites by private people. One day I received an E-mail from someone who had seen the extensive fetish links I run on my site, asking to be listed. He wrote:

**Don't forget about us! We're Balloon Buddies!**
**We have 255 members!**

This took my breath away (so to speak). I quickly went to the site and, lo and behold, there was an entire organization devoted to support and entertainment for people with a fetish for balloons. They exchanged messages, swapped pictures, and seemed to be an active little group.

Since then, I've been keeping an eye on balloon fetishism on the Net. As of this writing, there are about one hundred different Web sites devoted to it. Many of them are by men who have the fetish; but an equal number are by young women who evidently play with balloons for fun and profit. These clever young entrepreneurs (many of them claim to be coeds) make home videos of themselves bouncing around on big balloons, rubbing against them, popping them. Those fresh-faced beauties prancing around with balloons seem so strangely innocent.

Below, I am going to relate some more personal anecdotes about people with fetishes. These fetish tales may not reveal to you everything you would like to know about exactly how someone worships a fingernail, or why people who are perfectly normal in all other respects develop sexual kinks that most people would consider bizarre. The tales are here purely to open your mind to the incredible diversity of the human sexual imagination and to open your hearts to people whose sexual preferences and interests vary from yours.

## Bandages

This is a very brief tale, because language difficulties made it impossible to have more of a dialogue with this fellow. But one day, I received a brief note from a Japanese gentleman in somewhat tortured English. It went something like this:

**I am looking bandage fetich. Please help, are you finding any bandage fetich on Internet?**

I understood immediately that he was seeking a Web site devoted to his fetish, but suspected that his spelling was wrong and that he sought sites on bondage. I wrote back "bondage or bandage?" and received another short, hard-to-understand note that again said that he was seeking "bandage" sites.

I was still a bit confused, but saw that he had sent along a graphic image to explain. I opened up the file and looked at the picture and it all became quite clear. The picture showed a person (I can't say for sure that it was a woman, although I believe so) who was wrapped, head to toe, in surgical bandages, like the victim of a really bad car accident (except that there were no splints or casts to indicate any broken bones). She was completely covered in strips of white gauze, just two wide eyes and the tip of a nose peeping through.

This was new to me. I regretfully replied that I had not yet seen any Web sites devoted to it yet and would let him know if I found any. Not long afterwards, I found a set of similar images on one of the newsgroups devoted to fetish pictures. So I know he isn't alone. It's just a question now of someone building a Web site for this interest. Once someone does, I'm sure we'll discover there are hundreds of others like him.

## Bladder Enemas

I received an E-mail one day from an anonymous correspondent who identified herself as a woman and then asked, in very cautious, shy terms, whether I had ever heard of "bladder enemas" and whether I knew of any resources on the Internet where she could get information about how to do them safely.

I had to tell her that, unfortunately, I had no knowledge of this fetish and couldn't direct her to any resources. But, not wanting to leave her without hope, I went on to reassure her that while I hadn't heard of this particular fetish, I did know quite a few people had fetishes for medical scenes, and indeed I had an acquaintance who had a gynecological fetish. He liked to examine women closely, using speculums, and had developed quite a repertoire of gynecological techniques. Also, there are a number of men and women who are fascinated by urinary catheterization and incorporate that into their play.

I suggested she seek information under medical fetishes and catheters. She wrote back, apparently pleased with the advice, and we exchange a few more E-mails over the next few months.

Like a number of other women I've met with medical fetishes, she had, as a child, spent some time in and out of hospitals. The procedures, for better or worse, had taken on special meaning to her—again, something I've frequently observed in people with medical fetishes. For whatever reasons, these children begin to eroticize medical procedures—perhaps because the sheer vulnerability of the situation elicits unconscious arousal in them, or possibly because it is their first experience with adults who are doing what seem to be sexual things to them. As they grow to adulthood, some remember the procedures as erotic and long to re-create them.

In this woman's case, the bladder enema fit into a D&S context because of all the exposure and helplessness issues around this deeply intimate and controlling act. Over time, she found a dominant who was quite happy to experiment with her fetish, and they were beginning to make contacts with people who shared similar interests.

## Diapers

About ten years ago, I became online buddies with a woman who had a diaper fetish. I wouldn't characterize her as an infantilist, who is someone who enjoys dressing up in baby clothes and being treated as an infant. "Miriam" was very specifically turned on by the diapers themselves, and far less interested in giving up control or role-playing as a baby. She considered the diapers a very private fetish, and had only told a tiny handful of lovers about it, to varying degrees of success.

Miriam told me that simply being placed on a diaper was enough to bring her to the edge of orgasm, and that when a lover actually pinned it on her and she felt the cotton snugly pulled around her hips and between her legs, she could reach climax. She could also climax from peeing in the diaper—the warmth of the urine was apparently a fantastically erotic sensation for her.

There was more to her fetish than the erotic thrill. The diaper also made her feel safe and secure. As a harried professional in her daily life, she found that the diapers returned her to a safer, gentler, stress-free place when she was alone. Periodically, she would put on a diaper at the end of the day and wear it to sleep. She said that the diaper had an incredible calming effect on her and she would wake up the next day feeling emotionally refreshed and ready to face her adult world.

## Fantasy Creatures

One of my favorite fetish tales was told to me by a gay leatherman. "Sam" was a very experienced and adventurous bottom with a range of fetishes. He was always in search of new experiences with interesting new dominants.

Once, while visiting some leather friends in another city, Sam was told about a local top who shared his fetishes for heavy, immobilizing bondage, hoods, breath control, and rubber. At the bar that weekend, Sam's friends pointed the top out and recommended him as a safe, reputable player. It didn't take long for Sam to approach the man and strike up a conversation. Before long, he had finagled an invitation back to the top's dungeon so they could explore their shared fetishes together in private.

After arriving at the man's home, they went downstairs to his dungeon. The lighting was dim, and it got even darker for Sam as the man insisted on putting him in a blindfold before beginning their session. Sam was ready.

After blindfolding him, the top helped Sam climb into an elaborate full-body rubber suit of a type Sam had never worn before. It was made of extremely thick, rigid material. The suit had room for his legs and heavy sleeves for his arms as well. The man adjusted the suit, secured it on him, and finally, when Sam was completely immobilized, placed an enormous hood over Sam's head, completing the effect of total mummification.

Sam said it was one of the most exciting experiences of his life. Encased in the heavy rubber, he could not move; there were only two airholes by his nostrils that allowed him to breath. As he stood there helplessly immobilized, he could hear the dominant making love to his rubber-clad body. His own arousal intensified as it became clear that the dominant was *really* turned on, murmuring, grunting, panting, rubbing against the suit and ultimately climaxing.

Sam was still soaring with passion when the dominant pulled the hood off his head. Then, without warning, he removed Sam's blindfold. Sam blinked in surprise, his eyes adjusting to the gloom, and then, to his shock, he saw what looked like a huge grinning head in the dominant's arms. Indeed, it was a head: It was the head of Yogi the Bear. Apparently, the rubber suit which had brought them both so much erotic pleasure was an old Yogi the Bear costume, the kind used at a theme park to entertain children.

"I can't believe he took the blindfold off me and let me see it!" Sam later wailed. "Suddenly I realized he had been getting off on Yogi the Bear! It ruined everything for me."

Perhaps it ruined things for Sam, but it made for a great story!

## Fingernails

There was once an extremely gracious, gentle French business-man who had found his way from a small town in France onto the SM board I started on Compuserve. "Daniel" was in his fifties and for most of his life had struggled painfully with his need both to submit and to cross-dress. He and his wife shared a strict Roman Catholic background: In twenty-five years of marriage, they had never managed to have a civil conversation about his sexual needs. She was horrified when he tried to talk to her about his feminine side; she thought it was an abomination, that "a man should be a man."

Over time, Daniel retreated from her emotionally and was investing more and more time in his solitary fantasies. When he discovered the world of online kink, it was like a lifeboat to him in his sea of despair.

Perhaps because he'd been so alone with his fantasies for so many years—or perhaps because he was French—he had developed an extremely elaborate intellectual philosophy about sexuality and particularly female sexual dominance. He believed in female supremacy and envisioned a utopian universe where biological women ruled and biological men were transformed into females.

Daniel was a very interesting man indeed. Among his many kinks was an extreme fascination with long, sharp fingernails painted blood red. His idealized goddess had long claws, dripping with gore like some terrifying mythological siren. It seemed as if the very essence of cruel, devouring femininity was expressed by those ten tiny knives at the tips of his idol's fingers.

We lost contact eventually, but a couple of years ago I found a Web site devoted to "Gynocracy," or female superiority. The webmaster was apparently French, and there was something about the intellectual content that made me suspect "Daniel" had discovered yet another lifeboat online.

## Rubber/Latex

"Mark" was another person I met on Compuserve. He was a very intelligent, articulate man and we developed a friendly correspondence. Over the years, he told me a bit about himself and how he'd come to join my SM group. He was a retired government employee who had held a fairly important position for many years. Now he lived in comfortable retirement with his longtime wife. He had many children, and many more grandchildren, and he devoted most of his time to his family.

In recent years, though, he'd developed a tacit agreement with his wife: Simply, he had a certain amount of freedom to take off by himself, and she did not question what he did with that time.

Mark told me he had an intense, lifelong rubber fetish. Rubber and latex garments were at the core of his deepest sexual fantasies, along with fantasies of submission to goddess-like women. From time to time, when he could get away, Mark would take off and indulge these sexual needs.

Usually, he would take a trip for a weekend or a few days, and visit a dominatrix in another city who would dress him up in rubber or wear rubber herself. He also liked to attend a fetish ball that took place annually in New York City.

One year, he asked if I was planning to attend this ball. I was, and he quickly asked if I would be wearing rubber to the event. Well, a good rubber dress is an expensive proposition. At the time, I was teaching English at New York University and rubber dresses were not in the wardrobe budget. Mark told me that he had seen a red rubber dress in a window of a fetish boutique that he thought was absolutely gorgeous. His greatest desire was to see it on a woman he knew. He wondered whether I would consider wearing that dress if he bought it for me.

Men have bought me a lot of unique gifts over the years, but this was my first red rubber dress offer. I accepted, charmed by the idea and also grateful. I was sure it would be lovely. About a week later, a box arrived at my house and, sure enough, inside was a spectacular red latex dress.

Mark's face lit up when we met a few weeks later. When Mark asked me for a dance, I was more than happy to take his arm. I wore the skintight red rubber dress and Mark wore a head-to-toe latex outfit. As we danced, we made a lovely squeak together. Mark has told me many times since he will always cherish the memory of our romantic rubber dance and so will I.

## Vaccination Scars

Not very long ago, I received a letter from a very nice gentleman who wished to know whether others shared his erotic interest in vaccination scars. Although it made immediate sense to me that there would have to be people who would find those odd little dents on the upper arm sexy, I hadn't heard of this fetish. I planned to write him back but he beat me to it: The next day, I received another note from him, apologizing profusely. He was afraid he had offended me by revealing his fetish to me. What surprised me is that he felt so guilty about his fetish, which struck me as harmless and neither more nor less normal than any other sexual quirk.

I told him, as I've told so many others, that while I hadn't yet met anyone with his fetish, it was extremely unlikely that he was the only one who had it. He asked me whether I had a vaccination scar and I told him that I do, though it's quite small. I mentioned that I had older relatives who bore much larger scars from the vaccinations they'd received in earlier times.

Once he realized that I was not at all offended and, in fact, that I did not think it was any more or less weird than any other type of kink or fetish, he talked very enthusiastically about his interest. He was filled with questions and, mainly, I suppose, relief that someone did not see his desires as freakish. It empowered him to begin seeking friendships online with renewed hope.

## A CATALOGUE OF FETISHES

By now, you probably have figured out that the world of fetishes is virtually limitless. Anyone, at any time, can, for reasons that neither scientists nor psychologists can explain, develop an erotic fixation on an object or a part of a body.

Below is an incomplete list of types of fetishes, drawn from my research and from letters people have written to me over the years confiding their fantasies. In addition to inanimate objects and body parts, I also include types of people (such as amputees, obese people, or giants) who are the object of others' fetishistic fascination, as well as "action" fetishes (such as tickling or trampling).

If you don't see your fetish here, don't worry: Any such list would have to be incomplete. There are hundreds, if not thousands, of other fetishes that simply haven't been studied yet, or that have not yet made it into any of the sources that I drew on for this book. If you do have a fetish that doesn't show up on this list and you'd like to tell me about it, just visit my Web site (gloria-brame.com) and drop me a line. Who knows? By then, I may have already found a site on the Internet that caters precisely to your fantasies.

- *Adult Baby:* diapers, rubber pants/training pants, booties, bonnets, pacifiers, bottles, potties, rompers
- *Amputees;* also prosthetic limbs and devices
- *Animal Training (ponygirls and ponyboys, dog- or puppy-training):* dog dishes, cages, muzzles, leashes, collars, harnesses, reins, bits, saddles, spurs, dressage equipment (crops, whips, country bats), grooming equipment (curry combs and brushes)
- *Big or Fat People:* oversized breasts, disproportionately large (or small) sex organs, morbid obesity
- *Body Parts and Features (not covered in other categories):* knees, elbows, thighs, rectums, navels, necks, ears, facial expressions, hands, arms, enlarged muscles, surgical scars, knife wounds, keloids, vaccinations, burns, freckles, moles, tattoos, piercings, brands, cuttings
- *Clothing, Men's:* BVDs, jockey shorts, boxer shorts, socks, jockstraps, ties, suits, jackets, socks, work uniforms, tight jeans, wet jeans, leather chaps, suspenders, belts, hats, hand-

kerchiefs, overcoats, Speedos; also buttons, zippers, cufflinks, anything made of rubber, latex, pvc, spandex, plastic

• *Clothing, Women's:* angora sweaters, fuzzy sweaters, veils, hats, gloves, opera gloves, scarves, hoods, panties, white cotton panties, lace panties, girdles, slips, petticoats, brassieres, camisoles, garter belts, corsets, stockings, nylons, seamed stockings, panty hose, kneesocks, swimwear, bodysuits, catsuits, capes, maternity clothes, wedding gowns, jumpers, pleated skirts, school uniforms, nurse's uniforms, lab coats, nylon garments, wool garments, furs; also buttons, zippers, hooks and eyes, and any garments made of rubber, latex, pvc, spandex, plastic

• *Fantasy/Sacred Creatures:* aliens/ETs, robots, androids, demons, devils, mythological beasts, angels, fairies, vampires, werewolves, anime characters, American cartoon characters, inflatable dolls (sex toys), mannequins, half-human/half-animals, centaurs, satyrs, nymphs, Greek gods/goddesses, giants/giantesses, Amazons, Lilliputians

• *Feet and Legs:* big feet, small feet, clean feet, dirty feet, deformed feet, high arches, flat feet, heels, soles, callouses, corns, bound feet, toes, toenails, painted toenails, extra toes, missing toes, hammer toes, pigeon toes, bowlegs; also trampling, stomping, crushing, scissoring, kicking (see below for foot-tickling)

• *Fingernails:* long nails, clipped nails, filed nails, chewed nails, painted nails

• *Footwear:* boots (leather, rubber, fur), used boots, military boots, work boots, cowboy boots, wading boots, galoshes, wing tips, high heels, flats, sneakers, tennis shoes, Keds, ballet slippers, household slippers, ballet boots, stilettos, loafers, Oxfords, mary janes, patent leather shoes, go-go boots, thigh-high boots, shoelaces, lace-up shoes, shoes with buckles, cleats, sports shoes, clogs, mules, sandals, platforms, pumps, French heels, open-toed shoes

• *Hair:* beards, mustaches, chest hair, scalp hair, bald heads, body shaving, head shaving, sideburns, ponytails, braids, pigtails, long hair, gray hair, kinky hair, crew cuts, pubic hair; also hair combs, barrettes, hair ornaments, curlers, brushes, and combs

- *Headgear:* hats, hat brims, caps, hat decorations, construction hats, lace veils, tiaras, helmets, military hats
- *Masks*: half-masks, exotic (feathered) masks, costume masks, gas masks
- *Medical Equipment:* catheters, bedpans, hospital restraints, leg braces, wheelchairs, surgical bandages, plaster casts, medical devices, dental equipment, orthodontic braces, medical uniforms, surgical/latex gloves, speculums, enema bags, enema hoses, bardex nozzles, needles, hot-water bottles
- *Menstruation:* sanitary napkins, tampons, sanitary belts, menstrual rags
- *Messy/Gooey:* cream pies, shaving cream, mud
- *Midgets*
- *Military and Police Uniforms;* also Nazi uniforms
- *Plush Toys and Dolls* (including Barbie dolls and GI Joe)
- *Pregnancy:* lactating breasts, breast pumps, maternity clothes
- *Rubber, Latex, PVC, and Plastic:* any and all garments, sheets, pillowcases, rainwear, sleepwear, aprons, scuba gear, diving suits, hoods, masks, restraints
- *Smoking:* cigarettes, cigars, pipes, cigarette holders, celebrities and glamorous women who smoke, ashes, hot ash, role-playing as human ashtrays
- *Sports/Club Uniforms:* including all sports uniforms plus cheerleading uniforms, scouting uniforms
- *Tickling:* foot-tickling, underarm-tickling, tickling to the point of incontinence
- *Toy Balloons*
- *Wounds:* scars, piercings, deformities

CHAPTER EIGHT

# Role-Play and Lifestyle Relationships

This chapter takes a different approach to discuss a fantastically complex subject: role-playing and role-based lifestyle relationships. It consists of two sections. In the first, instead of responding to letters, I am providing a FAQ (an Internet term for "frequently asked questions") about lifestyle and role-playing, followed by my answers.

Section Two groups type of roles and relationships into basic, broad categories. The categories include brief descriptions of the common kinky roles people assume, as well as the kinds of scenarios, equipment, and clothes associated with these roles.

## SECTION ONE: ROLE-PLAY FAQ

### What Is Role-Play?

In the context of kinky sex, role-play is when people agree to step into roles or to express alternate personae in order to fulfill their sexual fantasies.

Role-playing takes many different forms. Some role-players take on a completely invented personality. They may imagine that they are warriors or pirates who conquer and torment their beautiful captives (a kind of role-play especially popular among folks who enjoy bondage). Or they may get turned on by a dominant who pretends to be a teacher or governess and disciplines the submissive who plays the role of a naughty child.

For others, role-playing is an opportunity to express a side of their identity that exists only in their bedrooms. They may even embellish on that secret self and endow it with a complete, albeit fantasy, identity. Some cross-dressers and even many dominants and submissives take this approach. They step into their roles for erotic purposes and return to their real-world identities when the fun and games are over.

## Aren't All Kinky People Just Playing Roles?

In a sense, we all play roles in life: "daughter," "son," "boss," "employee"—each expresses the different relationships we have with the people in our lives. With each role comes different feelings and responsibilities, and usually different behaviors and attitudes. But there is a difference between people who see BDSM and D&S as role-playing and people who see it as a lifestyle.

People who consider themselves role-players generally step in and out of their kinky roles according to their sexual appetites. They may really love to play the role of a ponyboy at a public club on weekends, for example, but just not want to do it every night at home. Or they may use role-playing mainly as sexual foreplay, acting out their fantasies with a partner until they are satisfied and then returning to their "normal" (non-kinky) relationship.

Those who identify as lifestylers will tell you that their kinky personae are real and legitimate expressions of their identities, and not role-play, which implies a time-limited or a fantasy scenario chiefly for the sake of erotic pleasure.

Lifestylers never step out of role because their roles and their relationships are inextricably intertwined. Just as a father's relationship with his children means a lifetime commitment to being a caretaker and protector, or as a teacher's relationship with her students is predicated on being an educator and leader in the classroom, a master's or mistress's relationship to a slave or submissive is based on a commitment to being the authority figure and mentor, both in the bedroom and outside it. Although they don't have SM sex all the time (even hard-core perverts do occasionally like to read books, see movies, and play computer games—why, some of us even have jobs!), lifestylers are always aware that one partner is in control and the other is under control.

## Are There Any Other Differences Between Role-Play and Lifestyle?

There are so many differences, they are too numerous to detail here. But in addition to the ones listed above, the most critical differences between role-playing and lifestyle have to do with the kinds of communications tools you use, the intimacy level you achieve, and often the amount of kinky sex you have.

To start backwards: Lifestyle SMers seem to indulge in sex more often than their vanilla or role-playing counterparts. The important distinction here, however, is that what constitutes "sex" for a lifestyler may not include intercourse or oral sex, but may focus instead on pain-play, bondage, head-play, and other erotic games. I've met many lifestyle couples who have some form of SM sex every day, or at least several times a week. On the other hand, most of the role-players I've known (with some notable exceptions) only have SM sex periodically or "episodically."

Another crucial distinction is that while role-play is, by its nature, time-limited, lifestyle is continual. The power dynamic is fixed between the partners, even if they conceal it from others. An example would be of a mistress telling her slave to call her for permission each time he needs to use the toilet, even if he's at work and must whisper. Lifestyle dominants have the authority to assert their power at any time.

Role-players may do this to escalate their arousal before a planned encounter. But once they step out of role, they do not presume that they wield authority over (or surrender it to) a play-partner. Instead, they obtain consent for each new SM interaction.

In terms of intimacy level, you can't have a lifestyle relationship with someone you just met. Lifestyle (like engagement and marriage) is a process that involves the gradual evolution of mutual trust, sexual harmony, and emotional commitment. Lifestyle implies a long-term and sometimes permanent commitment. The most intense (and intensely in love) lifestylers make unconditional lifetime commitments (with no possibility of separation or divorce).

But you can do role-play with someone you just met. Why? Because role-play doesn't require a long-term commitment; it just requires energy, imagination, desire, and, of course, consent.

If you are going to play a role with someone you don't know very well, safe words, contracts, and careful negotiation are your best protection against causing or receiving unintentional harm. But because lifestyle is predicated on the concept of a long-term process at a high level of intimacy, and since lifestyle often means a total power exchange, the above communications tools may become less important or irrelevant.

Lifestylers, for example, generally feel that safe words are artificial. In a lifestyle master/slave relationship, it is typical for the slave to grant his or her dominant blanket consent. This means that when a submissive makes a lifetime commitment to serve, he or she freely consents to a total surrender of power. This includes the sub's right to have a safe word, which gives the bottom or submissive ultimate control over a scene. The reason for this blanket consent is because, unlike role-players, they do not want to have the ultimate say-so about *anything*.

In return, lifestyle dominants take full responsibility for ensuring their submissives' well-being. If a dominant feels a safe word is the best way to gauge the submissive's reactions, then he or she will use one. But more commonly, lifestyle dominants prefer plain English to a code word. Like their submissives, they too feel that safe words undermine the reality of their power relationships. They treat SM sex as normal, nightly sex and not as an episodic experience.

Lifestylers, if they use a contract at all, tend to treat it much as a prenuptial agreement that sets out the parameters for a lifetime relationship. They also do not "negotiate" each scene because they do not see themselves as equals determining how they will interact once the play begins, but as dominants and submissives for whom the power roles are real at all times.

Role-players who are in committed, long-term (but not lifestyle) relationships may, over time, find that their communication is so good and their understanding of one another's needs so profound that they don't need to use safe words or contracts, either.

## Which Is Better: Lifestyle or Role-Play?

People ask me this all the time: Is one type of play better than another, or is one level of SM better than another?

Hear ye! Hear ye! When it comes to sex, *there is no such thing as "better." There is only "what's better for you."*

Fetishes, power relationships, and other kinky desires are universals. The desire for kinky sex cuts across all political, religious, economic, racial, and cultural lines. You can't expect all kinky people to share one point of view about what makes a kinky relationship perfect any more than you could expect all Americans to share one point of view about what makes a government perfect.

I recently spoke with a lovely, earnest submissive woman who was in deep conflict about her SM needs. She had been raised in a conservative, religious home. Her ideal was to meet "Mr. Right Master," marry, raise children, and lead a normal life together while enjoying an SM lifestyle relationship in private. She was disenchanted and ambivalent because every time she attended an SM party, or talked to people online, they pressured her to be more open about playing in public, doing SM at parties (often with strangers), and generally indulging in kink at a level she considered promiscuous. She worried that perhaps she wasn't really submissive, or submissive enough, because she found the whole concept of playing (as opposed to a lifetime commitment to one man) to be distasteful.

Clearly, she is still that nice, conservative, religious girl her parents raised. Where she went wrong was in trying to remake herself to fit some artificial model of "true submission." Being kinky does not mean that you give up who or what you were before, or that you transform your personality to fit some mold. There is no mold. Engaging in kink should be a matter of being true to yourself, as you are, and fulfilling your genuine desires. Your kinky persona should be a natural extension of your personality, not some act you put on so others will admire or approve of you.

My advice to this submissive was that she not compromise or give up her dream. Somewhere out there is a religious, conservative, monogamous dominant who would be more than happy to make babies with her and spank her—and not necessarily in that order, either.

If you choose to enter the Scene or explore a lifestyle relationship, your task is to learn what makes you happy and to take responsibility for your sexual well-being. Find out what particular sensations, scenarios, agreements, and commitments are the most fulfilling for you—personally or, if you're in a relationship, as a couple. What's right for others has nothing to do with what's right for you. Only you can decide that.

## Can Any Role Be Turned into a Lifestyle Relationship?

Just about, though there are roles that are difficult to maintain twenty-four hours a day. Infantilists may be able to sneak a diaper on under their suits, but they still can't sit at board meetings drinking from a bottle, nor would it be appropriate for them to vote "ga-ga" on whether or not the company should expand operations abroad. The same holds true for people who fantasize about being treated as animals, inanimate objects, hospital patients, and so on.

That said, they may all live the lifestyle at home. Some adult babies have relationships with their significant others where they remain in role all or most of the time, some rubber fetishists live in latex at home, and many transvestites make a lifestyle of cross-dressing.

One of the more interesting examples of role-play as lifestyle is the growing cult of kinky people who identify as "Goreans." Their relationships, social customs, mores, and sexual interactions are based on the GOR books by John Norman. Goreans assume the identities of the fictional characters and embrace the social philosophy behind Norman's fantasy world. They have, essentially, elevated role-play to a way of life.

## How Do I Know If I'm More of a Role-Player or More of a Lifestyler?

First, I'll tell you how you cannot know: You cannot know based on your fantasies. You can only know through experience.

In fantasy, we imagine all kinds of things, including scenarios that far exceed our ability either to cope with them emotionally or to act them out safely. Many people, in fantasy, dream of being fully owned slaves or captives. And most discover that, in reality, once the orgasm is over, they want to get back to reality without needing permission from someone else to eat a fudge sundae.

You will know if you are a lifestyler when you begin to gain some real-life experience. If you were cut out for lifestyle, experience with transient or purely role-play relationships will, over time, probably seem boring. They will not feel authentic enough to satisfy your deepest needs. On the other hand, if lifestyle is wrong for you, then you will find it difficult to stay in role for extended periods of time, and will long to get back to "reality" if it goes on for too long.

Another way to tell is not as reliable but is very telling. Simply put: If, after orgasm, your desire for kink is completely sated, and you don't feel submissive or dominant to the person you are with, chances are that lifestyle does not suit your temperament. If after orgasm, however, you cling to the feelings you just had and hope they never go away, chances are that, in the long run, role-play will not sustain you emotionally.

## SECTION TWO: ROUNDUP OF ROLES AND ROLE-BASED RELATIONSHIPS

While the list below may seem mind-boggling in its diversity, it actually only represents a fraction of the different types of erotic roles people play with one another. The human imagination is literally infinite.

I've created several broad categories of play. Very few people have had experience with them all, and some never experiment outside the particular category that turns them on the most. However, all of them are safely explored by millions of people every day. I've provided a concise definition of each category, listed the most popular types of role-play that fit the heading, and described typical scenarios, toys, and attire.

Finally, please remember that all of these roles are acted out by adults. You may personally feel uneasy about some of them, but all are based on consensual erotic agreements between adults. They do not involve children, animals, or anyone else who cannot give informed, explicit consent.

*Note:* N/A ("not applicable") is used wherever clothes or equipment are not necessarily part of the scene. However, creative players may improvise realistic wardrobes and equipment for any.

## Age-Play

One partner assumes the role of an older authority figure and the bottom or submissive takes on the role of the infant, child, or teenager.

### DADDY/BOY

Formal daddy/boy roles originated among gay leathermen, spread out into the non-kinky segments of the gay community, and have since been adapted by bisexual, lesbian, and heterosexual BDSMers. There are lesbian daddy/boy relationships (where both top and bottom assume male roles); male-dominant heterosexual daddy/boy relationships (where the femsub assumes the bottom "boy" role); and female-dominant heterosexual daddy/boy relationships (where the femdom assumes the top "daddy" role).

*Common Scenarios:* Daddy "raises" his boy; daddy presents his boy with his first leather clothes; daddy teaches boy about the birds and bees (and the whips and paddles); daddy punishes boy for infractions of rules; daddy whips boy, or takes him out to "the woodshed" (for discipline and control); daddy teaches boy how to please him sexually; boy serves as houseboy and takes care of all domestic chores as well as daddy's needs.

*Associated Equipment:* N/A.

*Associated Clothes:* A "boy" usually wears a locked collar. He may also (at SM parties) be scantily clad (a leather jockstrap and leather vest or harness is common). All biological females wear masculine clothes.

## MOMMY/BOY

This is a primarily heterosexual dynamic between a female dominant and a male submissive.

*Common Scenarios:* Mommy "raises" her boy; mommy spanks and otherwise physically punishes boy for bad behavior; mommy punishes boy by putting him in diapers, petticoats, and other humiliating (often feminizing) clothes; mommy teaches boy about his body; mommy teaches boy how to please a grown woman; mommy oversees boy's toilet habits.

*Associated Equipment:* N/A.

*Associated Clothes:* Short pants, Scout uniforms, diapers, petticoats, girl's clothes.

## DADDY/GIRL

In its most common form, this type of relationship implies male dominant/female submissive. Some lesbian tops also identify as daddies and enjoy playing with feminine "girl" partners.

*Common Scenarios:* Daddy spanks and punishes bratty girl; daddy pampers good girl and buys her toys; daddy worships girl because she is "his little princess"; daddy supervises girl's behavior and toilet habits; daddy dresses girl in childish clothes; daddy teaches girl about her body; daddy teaches girl how to please him sexually and otherwise.

*Associated Equipment:* N/A.

Role-Play and Lifestyle Relationships 173

*Associated Clothes:* Childish outfits (short skirts, anklets, mary janes, footed pajamas, rompers, jumpers, pinafores, rhumba panties, ribbons and bows, school uniforms, Scout uniforms).

## MOMMY/GIRL

My data on these types of relationships is limited to female dominants with cross-dressing male submissives and to lesbians.

*Common Scenarios:* Mommy "raises" girl; mommy selects girl's clothes and/or takes her shopping; mommy punishes girl for misbehavior; mommy nurtures and pampers girl; mommy takes care of all of girl's grooming needs; mommy teaches girl about her body; mommy teaches girl about the birds and the bees; mommy spanks and scolds girl for being a brat.

*Associated Equipment:* N/A.

*Associated Clothes:* The same types of clothing as for "daddy/girl."

## MOMMY OR DADDY/BABY

This form of age-play (infantilism) cuts across all orientations and is also the one most amenable to pansexual play, since infantilism only occasionally involves adult sexual activity. The focus here is to re-create the experience of infancy and early childhood (before toilet training) for the adult baby (AB).

Again, while I refer to parent/baby scenarios, some couples prefer to fantasize about other relatives or baby-sitters as the authority figure.

*Common Scenarios:* Parent keeps baby in diapers; parent feeds baby; parent cuddles and pampers baby; parent punishes naughty baby; parent makes baby soil diapers; parent makes baby be incontinent; parent helps baby to masturbate; parent makes sure baby's genitals are smooth (clean-shaven); parent shows baby how to make him or her feel good (sexually).

*Associated Equipment:* Rattles, bottles, pacifiers, baby toys, baby lotion, baby oil, baby powder; also adult or oversized cribs, high chairs, and playpens.

*Associated Clothes:* Diapers (ABs often have distinct preferences for either cotton or plastic), plastic pants, bibs, booties, bonnets, and any other baby clothes available in adult sizes.

### OTHER RELATIVES

Because some people are uneasy about parent/child age-play (which may feel too close to incest), imaginary aunts, uncles, cousins, or unrelated baby-sitters may substitute as authority figures who act as disciplinarians or take sexual advantage of "younger" relatives. These age-play relationships usually involve the same types of scenarios described above.

### BABIES TOGETHER

Sometimes because of a lack of a partner who will play the adult role, and sometimes because they simply enjoy it, two or more Adult Babies will play together. (Adult Babies may also switch roles, with one acting as parental authority. This is most likely to occur as a temporary means of satisfying needs in the absence of an adult-role partner, or in a monogamous relationship where both partners are ABs.)

*Common Scenarios:* Babies play with their toys together; babies soil their diapers together; babies makes big messes together; babies fight and bite and get rowdy together; babies suck their bottles together; babies explore each other's bodies; babies masturbate together.

*Associated Equipment:* Same as in mommy or daddy/baby.

*Associated Clothes:* Same as in mommy or daddy/baby.

### GOVERNESS OR TEACHER/STUDENT

The dominant plays the role of an educator who closely supervises and disciplines student. Punishment is for the student's "own good," often to improve his or her "moral character."

*Common Scenarios:* Governess punishes her ward for disobedience; governess monitors her ward's personal hygiene; schoolmistress or schoolmaster punishes student for failing to study; nonpainful punishments appropriate to schoolchildren (repetitive writing exercises, standing in a corner, scolding, humiliation); corporal discipline (particularly spanking, caning, and paddling).

*Associated Equipment:* Paddles, canes, belts, rulers, and other implements associated with old-fashioned school punishments.

*Associated Clothes:* Victorian garb or other conservative clothing for the dominant; otherwise, no specific attire.

### FRATERNITY HAZINGS

Generally, most common among gay, bisexual, or bi-kinky men, the participants see themselves as young, wholesome, clean-cut, college-aged buddies. Switching and group-play is common.

*Common Scenarios:* Spanking and paddling; hazings (though still with a strong emphasis on paddling); discipline by a housemaster or older student for bad-boy behavior.

*Associated Equipment:* Paddles and other spanking devices.

*Associated Clothes:* Street clothes suitable to young men, underwear (BVDs, jockeys, jockstraps, athletic socks).

## Animal-Play

A type of role-play in which the bottom or submissive is treated and trained as an animal or pet.

### DOG TRAINER AND DOG/PUPPY

*Common Scenarios:* Feeding the dog from a dog dish; leading the dog by collar and leash; paper training or "walking" the dog outdoors; refusing the dog permission to speak English and instead making the dog bark, whimper, beg, and so on to communicate needs; teaching the dog basic commands, including "fetch"; training the dog to perform pet tricks; having the dog lick and lap at body parts (oral sex); petting, pampering, playing with, and grooming dog.

*Associated Equipment:* Any and all types of dog equipment (including dog treats) available at a pet shop.

*Associated Clothes:* Dogs are kept naked. Trainers wear regular street clothes.

### PONY-PLAY

Roles include trainer or rider and horse or pony.

*Common Scenarios:* Harnessing (and/or saddling) the pony; teaching the pony to prance, trot, gallop, and perform tricks.

*Associated Equipment:* Tack gear and equestrian supplies such as whips, crops, bats, curry combs, grooming brushes; also horsetails (for anal insertion) and lassoes.

*Associated Clothes:* For the top only: English riding uniform and equestrian boots or western boots, spurs, chaps, leather vests, western shirts, jeans, cowboy hats. For the bottom: saddles, bits, harnesses, reins, and headdresses.

### HANDLER/FARM ANIMAL

*Common Scenarios:* Cow is milked vigorously (the breasts with females; the penis or nipples with males); pig is treated contemptuously and subjected to torture and degradation.

*Associated Equipment:* Any farm equipment that can be safely adapted to human play.

*Associated Clothes:* None, though the bottom is usually kept naked.

## Torturer/Captive Prisoner

These fantasies center around images of forced captivity. The top (or dominant) is a sadist who mercilessly torments the bottom (or submissive), often pushing limits both in terms of pain-play and mind-play.

### PRISON GUARD/PRISONER

*Common Scenarios:* Humiliating physical inspections (including examination of body cavities); rape and forced sex; beatings and verbal abuse; rigid bondage; imprisonment in a cell block or cage; solitary confinement. In other words, a typical day in prison.

*Associated Equipment:* Handcuffs, fetters, chains, pain toys.

*Associated Clothes:* Guard uniforms and prison uniforms.

## INQUISITOR OR INTERROGATOR/VICTIM

*Common Scenarios:* Interrogator tortures victim to extract confessions; bastinado (beatings on the soles of the feet).

*Associated Equipment:* Extreme bondage and pain toys, including electrotorture devices and large-scale equipment.

*Associated Clothes:* N/A.

## MILITARY PERSONNEL/VICTIM

*Common Scenarios:* Boot camp fantasies, with drill sergeants and others terrorizing young recruits into strict obedience; uniformed personnel raping helpless victim; cops or military police making brutal arrest; Nazi officer abusing prisoner/whore.

*Associated Equipment:* Bondage and pain toys.

*Associated Clothes:* Uniforms, uniforms, and more uniforms!

## Caught and Punished

These fantasies involve the bottom (or submissive) partner being caught doing something naughty or bad, and the top (or dominant) disciplining the person (usually with spanking and paddling), demanding sex in exchange for silence, and otherwise "forcing" the bottom to accept punishment.

## Authority Figure/Misbehaving Adult

These fantasy roles take hundreds of different twists in the human imagination. Not all of them depend on the top taking on an authoritarian role; in some scenarios, the person giving punishment is an equal who has gained an "unfair" advantage by discovering that someone is hiding a "terrible secret."

*Common Scenarios:* Authority figure finds slut masturbating and punishes slut (usually with spankings); authority figure finds naughty boy (or girl) looking at X-rated materials and either punishes or demands sexual services; social equal (neighbor, coworker) threatens misbehaving adult with exposure and "forces" him or her to accept humiliating punishment (or demands sex); boss discovers company crime by employee and threatens to fire unless employee agrees to humiliating punishment (or demands sex).

*Associated Equipment:* N/A.

*Associated Clothes:* N/A.

## Gender-Play

(Also see "Age-Play," as some transgendered roles revolve around age-play scenarios.)

*Common Scenarios:* Dressing up in opposite-sex clothing; being "forced" (by a dominant) into opposite-sex clothing.

*Associated Equipment:* N/A.

*Associated Clothes:* Any opposite-sex clothing.

## Goddess Worship

This pagan-inspired form of role-play is based on the belief that women are the human incarnations of world-shaping goddesses, and that dominant women have achieved the spiritual and sexual enlightenment necessary to manifest divine characteristics. Goddess worshippers cut across gender lines, but are most commonly heterosexual men.

*Common Scenarios:* Abject worship (including foot worship and body worship); crawling, groveling, and verbally exalting the goddess; accepting punishment and torture to satisfy the goddess's dark side; making offerings (sexual, monetary, and otherwise) to the goddess in hopes of gaining her attention.

*Associated Equipment:* N/A.

*Associated Clothes:* None, though the goddess may choose to enhance her aura with flowing garments, extravagant jewels, and loosened hair.

## Hospital Fantasies

*Common Scenarios:* Doctor, nurse, or other medical personnel subjects patient to humiliating inspections; painful or humiliating medical procedures (may involve neuro-wheels, speculums, catheters); enemas; temperature-taking with rectal thermometer; diapering or supervised urination and defecation; forced sex; body-shaving and sponge-bathing.

*Associated Equipment:* Hospital equipment, including (but not limited to) bedpans, enema kits, catheters, restraints, traction devices, leg braces, examination tables (sometimes with stirrups), thermometers and tongue depressors, forceps.

*Associated Clothes:* Scrubs, nursing uniforms, and other medical uniforms for the dominant; revealing pajamas for the patient.

# Owner/Inanimate Object

*Common Scenarios:* Human ashtray passively accepts hot ash dropped by owner (usually smoking cigar); footstool crouches on all fours while dominant rests feet on its back; table bends over (while standing) to hold ankles, so dominant may rest plate or glass on surface of its back.

*Associated Equipment:* N/A.

*Associated Clothes:* N/A.

# CHAPTER NINE

# Transgenderism: The Second Self

## WHAT'S IN A GENDER?

*My fiancé is educated, successful, and loves children. Perfect marriage material—or so I thought. This past weekend, I caught him wearing my panties! It led to a terrible fight. He told me that he is a transvestite. He says he has been cross-dressing his whole life and he asked me if I will accept him as he is. His abnormal needs shocked me. I told him I will only marry him if he promises never to do it again. He said he will try. Do you think marriage will make a real man of him? Should I make him get counseling first?*

In order to understand transgenderism, you have to throw away the tired notion that there is such a thing as a "real man" or a "real woman." "Real," in this context, implies that anyone who doesn't meet the mythical ideal of masculine (or feminine) perfection is sexually inadequate. This is untrue. While it sometimes seems as if men and women are so different they come from different planets, the fact is that the lines between male and female behavior are often blurry.

Science has not been able yet to prove, with certainty, that there is a biological basis for behaviors we have traditionally considered masculine or feminine. Scientists have identified some differences in the structure of male and female brains, but they do not yet understand the full meaning of these differences. Even where they can account for general trends in aptitudes, there remain so many questions, and so many exceptions, that the debate is open. Some well-touted cases have turned out to be scientifically hollow; others have produced results that are open to interpretation.

It would be wonderful, from a sexological perspective, if we had hard data to explain why some people are more masculine or feminine than others. Scientists have speculated for over a century about the possibility of a genetic basis for homosexuality, transgenderism, fetishism, and other minority sexual identities. But the proof does not yet exist. So, for now, we must rely on what we know from anecdotal data and our own observations.

We know, for example, that societies create idealized models of male and female identity. We know that children are taught to conform to those models: We encourage boys to play at being soldiers and fighters and girls to play at being mothers and homemakers. We know that adults honor the social ideal and pressure those around them to do the same.

We also know that, despite all this, people seldom fit the ideal. Most of us fluidly combine traditional male and female qualities. It's typical for men to possess allegedly feminine qualities (tenderness, sensitivity, dependency, vulnerability, submissiveness) and for women to express allegedly masculine ones (aggressiveness, insensitivity, independence, strength, dominance). Typing certain feelings and behaviors as uniquely masculine or feminine is in itself a large part of the problem. It makes people believe there is such a thing as a "real man" or a "real woman" when, in fact, gender identity is simply not that black and white.

Finally, we know that even the most rigidly conformist cultures produce transgenderists (TGs)—people who "cross gender" either by living out an opposite-sex role or by medically undergoing a sex change. In effect, TGs have two gender identities: their biological identity and an opposite-sex identity that may be less intense than, equal to, or more intense than their biological identity.

Transgenderism has been widely documented throughout the world, in all cultures. There is documentation of transvestism dating to the Egyptian dynasties. King Tut's father, the revolutionary pharaoh Akhenaton, was reputed to occasionally dress in women's garb. The Roman emperor Nero, guilt-stricken over killing his wife in a fit of rage, compelled a young man to dress up as his dead bride and married the transvestite in a bizarre public ceremony.

In some Native American cultures, transgenderists were revered as spiritual figures. Transvestites (young men dressed as women) have been employed at brothels throughout the Middle East and Orient for millennia. During the American Civil War, hundreds of women dressed as men and served in the Union Army, perhaps taking inspiration from Joan of Arc, who also cross-dressed for political reasons. American legend Annie Oakley is remembered as the girl who could shoot like a man. But Ms. Oakley didn't just shoot like a man: she acted and lived as one in all respects and would, today, be acknowledged as a transgenderist. Simply put, there has never been a time or place in history when people did not wear the clothes and affect the mannerisms of the opposite sex.

While drag queens and postoperative transsexuals appear regularly on television nowadays, they are not representative of the vast majority of TGs. Because of bigotry against people who cross the gender line, a transvestite or preoperative transsexual is far more likely to hide in the shadows of a dark bar than to be flaunting him- or herself in front of camera lights.

One of the most fascinating stories of our time is that of the late jazz musician Billy Tipton. Until his death in 1989, Tipton lived and worked as a man. When his clothes were removed after his death, it was revealed that he was in fact a biological female—news that came as a stunning surprise to his children and ex-wives. The mystery of how Tipton managed to fool his intimates for all those years went to the grave with him, leaving us to speculate how many other Billy Tiptons live quietly among us, guarding their gender secret.

A person who has two gender identities cannot be changed by marriage or by counseling. Transgenderism is at the heart of an individual's identity. A competent therapist will not attempt to tamper with that identity but will instead help the TG to cope with his or her situation. A TG may repress his or her need for a time, but that won't make the need go away. More likely, it will drive the person to act out his or her needs in secrecy.

Couples counseling may help lovers deal better with transgenderism, but if you are expecting your partner's needs to change, you will be disappointed. If change is to come, it will have to come from the partner who is hostile to or otherwise uneasy with transgenderism. Learning to relax some of your attitudes about what a man or woman "should" be and to educate yourself on the realities of transgenderism are the first steps.

If someone you love is transgendered, and you, for whatever personal reasons, cannot accept this, even after counseling, it's best to make a clean break. Asking someone to shut off a fundamental component of his or her identity is essentially dooming a person to unhappiness. Worse, it will usually drive a person to lead a double life, filled with lies and deceptions. Sooner or later, with you or without you, a TG will need to release the opposite-sex identity within.

## TRANSVESTITE OR TRANSSEXUAL?

Most people are able to accommodate male and female characteristics within themselves. Women can show courage without feeling less feminine, and a tenderhearted man is sometimes considered more masculine than a macho iceberg. Many of us can also wear opposite-sex clothes, either as a joke or an adventure, without feeling that it says anything about us, except that we're bold and experimental.

Transgenderists come from a different place. Their male and female sides are often (though not always) split into distinctly different compartments, and are expressed through separate personalities. In other cases, there may be an absence of boundaries between masculine and feminine, so that the TG is fundamentally androgynous.

Transgenderism includes two separate but related phenomena: transvestism (or cross-dressing) and transsexualism.

The most visible type of transvestite (TV) is the drag queen, a gay man who wears flamboyant costumes and performs stage shows. Drag queens are usually performance artists (even if their only audience is a mirror). They generally don't derive sexual pleasure from the clothes, though they may enjoy having sex with their male lovers while cross-dressed.

Overall, drag queens are only a tiny percentage of the total transvestite population. Clinical research suggests that between 0.1 and 1 percent of American men are cross-dressers. Of this number, only roughly 2 percent of men who cross-dress are gay; the other 98 percent are heterosexual. My own research suggests that many self-identified heterosexual TVs have bisexual fantasies, or have had bisexual encounters. The number one reason they give is that they crave to understand how their biological opposite feels in bed.

According to a 1993 CIA report on transgenderism, one in 30,000 men and one in 100,000 women are transsexual. In 1998, the International Foundation for Gender Education cited data that between 50,000 and 75,000 people in the United States currently live, work, and dress as members of the opposite sex.

Cross-dressing is about transformation. It releases the TV from the constraints of their biological sex into the power, freedom, and eroticism that belonging to the opposite sex represents in the TV's mind. For male-to-female TVs in particular, every aspect of the gender transformation may be intellectually intriguing, sexually thrilling, and psychologically liberating.

The vast majority of cross-dressers are male-to-female (biological men who dress as women). Unlike the m-t-f TV, female-to-male cross-dressers tend, more often than not, to be gay. The lesbian butch is a common example of a biological female who wears masculine clothes and projects a male identity. In leather culture, some butches prefer to be called daddy, sir, or master by their submissives and slaves. There are also lesbian submissives who dress as young men and live out a daddy/boy relationship with a butch dominant. Some female-to-male cross-dressers eroticize masculine attire, particularly denim, leather garments or footwear, and military uniforms.

Wearing opposite-sex attire (as well as wigs or cosmetics) is key for m-t-f TVs. They may derive erotic satisfaction from the clothing itself. On one end of the range you'll find people who only want to wear a few opposite-sex garments (typically, a skirt, or panties, or stockings and high heels). At the other end are those who painstakingly reproduce, down to the last polished toenail and false eyelash, a flawless simulation of femininity. They spend hours on manicures, clothing selection, hairstyling, and application of cosmetics. Few biological women invest as much time in—or get as much pleasure from—primping.

The dressing may take on ritual aspects. There may be specific garments (such as seamed stockings, fuzzy sweaters, or corsets) that play an almost fetishistic role in the dressing-up. Some TVs are so intent on complete transformation that they will take pregnancy tests and use feminine douches and deodorants, undergo electrolysis, pretend to get menstrual periods, and even wear sanitary devices (not always in the most sanitary places, either—tampons really only fit comfortably into one orifice on a man's lower body). I've met a handful who wore the wedding gowns when they married their understanding spouses. Needless to say, every minute detail of these processes may bring a TV a special thrill.

Erotic pleasure, however, is not the only—or even most important—reason that TVs cross-dress. The transformation process brings them sheer psychological relief. A transvestite, essentially, has a second opposite-sex self bottled up inside, and if that identity is not expressed, a transvestite may become stressed, depressed, dysfunctional, desperate, and even suicidal. Opposite-sex clothes or other forms of expression of an opposite-sex identity (such as role-play) are necessary to a transvestite's mental health.

Transvestites do not wish to *become* the opposite sex in reality. Their other self is an alternate aspect of their personality, not their entire identity. They may fantasize about belonging to the opposite sex, and they certainly need to act out their fantasies, but they also enjoy certain aspects of their biological sex. Butch women, for example, are usually quite happy to be women under the clothes, and male-to-female transvestites usually appreciate the social and economic privileges of being men.

A small percentage of m-t-f TVs hover ambivalently at the border between TV and TS—they may, for example, take herbal formulations of female hormones (available at holistic health shops) in hopes of bulking up their bustline. They are not, however, prepared to make a full-scale commitment to changing their sex (through implants and other surgical procedures) and, despite their explorations, may never be.

Unlike transvestites, transsexuals feel so strong an affinity with the opposite sex that they do wish permanently to change their bodies. From earliest childhood, they feel estranged from, confused by, and sometimes disgusted by their sexual equipment. For the TS, dressing in the clothes of the opposite sex isn't about transforming into another self; it's about expressing one's true identity. The clothing is a part of it but never an end in itself (as it may be for a TV).

Transsexuals fall into two basic groups: preoperative and postoperative. A pre-op TS may dress and live as a member of the opposite sex, but retains the genitalia he or she was born with. A post-op TS has undergone sex-change surgery and is now a member of the opposite sex.

Transsexuals, as a rule, believe themselves to be victims of a biological mistake: They believe the reproductive systems they were born with are, in a real sense, birth defects. (Indeed, many transsexuals say they feel disgusted by their genitals or breasts for this reason.) Science may ultimately prove that their feelings have a medical basis. Clinical research into transsexualism tentatively suggests that a kind of chemical accident occurs during pregnancy that causes people to be born transsexuals. It's possible that a sudden and intense hormonal imbalance in the mother's womb may create a genetic anomaly in the fetus. As yet, we don't know this for sure, but the preliminary data is promising.

While transsexuals may feel that they are really members of the opposite sex "trapped" in the wrong body, not all of them want to undergo sex-change operations (known as "sexual reassignment surgery" or SRS). Actually, it's something of a misnomer to call it a sex-change operation since it actually requires a lengthy series of surgeries to complete the process. Biological men who wish to become biological women have breast implants (or get injections of silicone), undergo complete castration (penis and testicles) and removal of internal male reproductive equipment, and endure plastic surgery to form a vagina. Amazingly, surgeons are able to create remarkably real vaginas, which are sensitive to sexual stimuli. In some cases, a postoperative m-t-f TS will be able to experience orgasm with the new genitalia; none, however, can bear children. Science can build an astonishingly authentic fascimile of a vagina, but not of a womb.

Most m-t-f transsexuals also need a range of cosmetic surgeries to feminize their features. These include jaw reduction, removal of the male "Adam's apple," and so on. They also require permanent hair removal, typically through a long series of painful and costly visits to an electrolysist.

Biological women who wish to become biological men have their breasts removed and undergo hysterectomies, and their vaginas are closed off. A realistic penis, however, is still beyond the art and craft of the surgeon. Medical technology has not yet developed a way to create the muscles or nerve tissues necessary to give f-t-m transsexuals a real experience of having a penis. They are instead equipped with grafted skin, shaped like a tube to accommodate a prosthetic device, which inflates. It gives the appearance of an erection and allows them to penetrate their partners. However, this penis doesn't function like a real one. Female-to-male transsexuals cannot achieve orgasm by stimulating the medical miracle between their legs (through intercourse or otherwise), nor can they produce semen.

While SRS is so arduous that one might wonder whether it's worth it, for some transsexuals it seems to be the only acceptable solution. There are wonderful success stories of people who have made a satisfying transition from one sex to the other, and who lead happier lives in their new bodies.

Unfortunately, this isn't true for everyone. Many postoperative transsexuals have discovered, to their despair, that the emotional scars of growing up TS in our society are not healed by surgery. In some cases, the surgery is even more traumatic to them than their transsexualism. Some regret their decision. A few have wanted to reverse the process later on. Sadly, as difficult as it is to go from one sex to another, it is even more difficult to go back. Once a man has been castrated, he will never again have normal male genitals. Female-to-male post-ops can no longer bear children.

Because of these many problems, a high percentage of transsexuals only take their biological transformation partway. They may take hormones prescribed by their doctors to help them achieve cosmetic changes (these would include hormones to help male-to-female transsexuals develop breasts, and hormones to help female-to-male transsexuals develop more body hair and thicker builds). Hormone therapy is risky and requires close medical supervision. Over time, it produces hermaphrodites: people with the secondary characteristics of both sexes. Popular terms for these medically engineered hermaphrodites are "she-males" or (more vulgarly) "chicks with dicks."

Although she-males combine male and female charms, they aren't true hermaphrodites, because they possess only one set of reproductive organs, either male or female. I do know one f-t-m TS who had her breasts removed and acquired a grafted penis but also retained her vagina. Her name is Linda/Les and she was partnered for years with porn diva Annie Sprinkle. The couple made a performance art of this unusual choice by doing stage shows in which Annie, dressed like a naughty nurse, soberly explained the differences between pre-op and post-ops transsexuals, using Linda/Les as the primary visual aid. When Linda/Les lowered her/his pants, it was indeed very/visual.

Presumably Linda/Les wanted to keep her vagina so she could continue to enjoy direct sexual pleasure (and orgasms). Or maybe she had issues with commitment. In any case, she is the only one I know of personally who has made this choice, though I suspect there must be others.

While true hermaphroditism is rare, it is widely documented in the medical literature. Usually, one set of genitals is more obvious than the other. The second set of organs is sometimes tiny or nonfunctional. Parents of hermaphrodites may attempt to raise the child according to the way he or she looks rather than how she or he feels. This can cause more harm than good to the child.

The best approach is to take the child for genetic testing. Tests will reveal the person's chromosomal makeup. Once the doctors know whether the child is genetically male or female, and can predict how he or she will mature in later years, surgery may be recommended to forestall future problems. Depending on the child, the operation may be minor or not so minor. In either case, it should not be viewed as sex-change surgery but as corrective surgery that rights one of nature's wrongs.

A physican friend once told me about the most unusual case of hermaphroditism that I've come across in my research. A couple brought their eldest daughter to the hospital to see specialists. She was already seventeen but her breasts were underdeveloped and she had not yet begun to menstruate. Doctors were soon surprised to find that while the girl had what appeared to be a normal vagina, she did not have a womb. The vagina led nowhere—it was simply a kind of gratuitous opening. She also had a tiny penis hidden under the vaginal lips.

They asked to examine the girl's two younger sisters and discovered that all three of them were identically formed. Upon genetic testing, they determined that, chromosomally speaking, all three girls were actually boys.

To the distraught parents, the doctors explained that they could remove the tiny, incomplete penises that were somewhat hidden inside the girls' labia. Their breasts would always remain small, but the girls—who had been raised as females and were happily feminine both in appearance and behavior—would be able to lead fairly normal lives as women. Sadly, though, none of them would ever be able to bear children.

## COMMON CONCERNS OF TVS AND SOME ADVICE

Because transvestism and transsexualism are such awesomely complex phenomena, which take on so many different forms, it would be impossible to list every single problem and challenge that transgenderists face. In this section, I focus instead on the most common problems that the largest percentage of TGs—male-to-female cross-dressers—encounter in their daily lives.

### Divorce and Loss of Children

Transvestites often end up with partners who are hostile to their second self. They live in perpetual fear of discovery and often restrict their cross-dressing to times when they are out of town on business or have total privacy at home. They believe, with some justification, that their spouses may divorce them. Equally anguishing is the possibility that attorneys will use their cross-dressing as a weapon in a custody trial, and convince the court that transgenderists are unfit parents (an argument judges frequently accept prima facie despite the lack of proof).

If you are permanently partnered with someone who doesn't know that you cross-dress, or who is hostile to your gender duality, investigate couples counseling as soon as possible. Seek out a therapist who has had experience dealing with cross-dressers before. It is crucial that you find someone who takes a sympathetic attitude towards gender issues so that the therapy does not become about "curing" you, but instead about helping you and your partner develop strategies to cope with your needs.

If divorce is already on the horizon and you are worried about custody issues, hire a competent lawyer as soon as humanly possible. Don't be embarrassed to explain the full situation to your lawyer: He or she has definitely heard worse and, besides, lawyers are bound by confidentiality. Do not delay to prepare a legal strategy to protect your rights and your children's future.

You can find support, guidance, and advice on family issues through TG organizations. If you have Internet access, visit my TV/TG links page (gloria-brame.com/tvtgts.htm) and surf from there to dozens of excellent resources to help you cope. You don't need to face it all alone.

## Destruction of Career

A cross-dresser I met some years ago worked in a very high-profile job in the media. He had a recurrent nightmare in which he went out in drag and was suddenly blinded by camera flashes as his colleagues swooped down on him, making him their headline of the day. He would wake up in a state of terror, vowing never to go out in drag again—a vow that only lasted as long as he was able to repress his need.

Unfortunately, he was not being unduly paranoid. There is so much ignorance about cross-dressing that TVs may be at risk if their boss or a competitive colleague learns of their secret identity. In some states, employers have the law on their side if they decide to fire you for it.

The best advice is not to talk about your sex issues at the office. Next, don't have affairs with coworkers who might talk about it. For the most part, the people you work with don't need (or want) to know about your sex life. This is just plain common sense, applicable to all adults. Keep your sex life in the sexual realm and your professional life professional and you should do fine.

Some people feel a moral or political obligation to make their sexual orientation known in the workplace. That is a matter of personal conscience. In some respects, I wish everyone had the courage to be open about their sexual identities—then "unusual" desires wouldn't seem so unusual. But since most people play it safe, I advise you do the same. Don't take risks if you can't face their possible consequences.

### Social Rejection and Derision

Despite the strides women have made socially and economically since the 1970s, women are still viewed as the weaker sex. For a man to need to wear a dress or to have obviously feminine attributes suggests to a lot of people that he must therefore be weak too. While TVs may have a female identity, they still have enough of a masculine one to have a bit of the old male ego.

This may partly explain why the majority of male-to-female transvestites who visit professional dominatrices are known to be overachievers in traditionally macho fields where they are constantly called upon to prove that they've got what it takes. Never mind that their what-it-takes is encased in silk panties. Those who see the suit on top seldom have any idea that there are panties underneath. When they do, they may make cruel barbs and ugly jokes at the TV's expense.

While transgendered people are as likely as any other oppressed minority to combat stress with laughter, they are also (like any other oppressed minority) sensitive to cutting remarks from insensitive boobs. If bullies taunted them when they were young, the lasting hurt can make any joke very difficult to take, no matter its source.

## Gender Dysphoria

Gender dysphoria is the clinical term to describe the unhappiness and, at times, severe depression that many TGs go through when they have a lot of unresolved issues and frustrations about their gender identity.

If TGs do not have satisfying outlets for their needs, the tension between their dual identities can grow unbearable. One cross-dresser I knew regularly went through purges. Just as bulimics binge one day and starve the next, he would periodically throw his frilly things into the incinerator in shame and disgust, only to invest wildly in new clothes when the need again grew too strong to resist.

Transgendered personalities can become so stressed out that they feel torn apart. Under the strain of repression and frustration, their fantasies may reach new extremes, confusing them even further.

Strive for a balance by finding satisfying, acceptable, consensual outlets for your needs. Meditation may help, as will the support of peers. If you are losing sleep, having difficulty concentrating, or finding it difficult to keep your personal life and career afloat, don't hesitate to get counseling. Dysphoria can be treated. Purging will only lead to a new wardrobe.

## QUICK QUESTIONS FROM PARTNERS OF TVS

I get a lot of E-mail from the partners (usually wives or girl-friends) of m-t-f transvestites. Their concerns range from relationship issues to practical matters. Here is a brief compendium of some of the most interesting and poignant questions I've been asked.

**Question:** *My husband and I are expecting our first child. I am worried that somehow his cross-dressing will have a negative impact on family life. Up until now, we were alone, but with a baby on the way, I* *worry about it. Can he be a good father if he keeps on cross-dressing, or should I beg him to stop for the sake of our future family?*

**Answer:** A person's sexual orientation has absolutely no effect on his or her parenting skills. Neither do people inherit their parents' sexual eccentricities.

On the whole, TVs are very family-oriented. If your husband is a responsible and caring individual, then he will do just fine. Because m-t-f TVs do have a feminine side, and are thus finely attuned to feminine emotions, many TVs may bring a special maternal tenderness to their parenting.

The only time a partner of a TV should feel concerned is when the clothes and role-playing seem more important to a cross-dresser than their personal relationships and responsibilities. If your partner fulfills his commitments and spends quality time (and plenty of it) with you and your children, then there is no reason whatever to make him cut back on his cross-dressing. He's got it all under control.

**Question:** *Sometimes I let my husband wear my nightgown to bed at night. It used to bother me but now I don't mind. It makes him so happy. The other night, though, he said something strange after we made love. He said he felt like he'd had a lesbian experience. Does he think I'm a lesbian because I let him wear my nightgown, and that means I want to be with another woman? If that's what he meant, the gowns are going straight up to the attic!*

**Answer:** Don't pack just yet.

The lesbian your husband was referring to was himself, not you.

Because most male-to-female TVs are heterosexual, even when cross-dressed they wish to make love with women. But they don't see it as a typical male/female encounter (which, obviously, it is not if he is wearing your nightgown). Instead, a TV will fantasize that he's having a lesbian affair.

This does not, by any means, imply that a TV actually believes his wife or girlfriend is lesbian. It's simply his way of sustaining the fantasy that he is a biological female.

**Question:** *My lover likes to cross-dress and I enjoy it fine. Recently, he told me he would like me to force him into the clothes. I don't understand. How can you force someone into doing something you know they like?*

**Answer:** Forced feminization is an extremely popular fantasy among TVs. The basic scenario is that a powerful woman coerces a man, often as a form of punishment, into embarrassing feminine clothing. Coercion fantasies (which are discussed in chapter 5 on bondage) require role-play. In reality, both partners have consented to the scene, but in their respective roles one is the aggressor and the other her helpless victim.

As with bondage, the submissive partner who is coerced into opposite-sex clothes feels liberated by his lack of options. That is why such forced-feminization fantasies often involve an angry wife giving her husband an ultimatum ("either wear this corset for the next two weeks or I'll leave you!") or a female authority figure (a boss, a teacher, an aunt) discovering him in some shameful predicament and cross-dressing him as punishment. In such a scenario, he is no longer responsible for wearing the clothes: It is that cruel vixen (his understanding partner, in other words) who has forced him into this humiliating circumstance.

This type of play isn't for everyone, but for those who like D&S with their cross-dressing, forced feminization opens the door to dozens of pleasurable variations.

**Question:** *I was willing to accept it when my husband confessed he was a cross-dresser. But when he showed me how he looked in drag, I was stunned. He looks better than me. Now I feel even worse than before. I don't want to be seen in public with my husband when he looks prettier than me.*

**Answer:** There is no easy answer to such a conundrum. Most women find it challenging enough to go out with girlfriends who look better; when your man looks cuter in a dress, it's got to be tough on the feminine ego. But the bottom line is this: Are you going to let your vanity stop you from having a good time?

If you really have a problem with such an issue, tell your partner about it and let him reassure you of his love and attraction for you. Just as you are giving him a tremendous gift by accepting him for who he is and encouraging him to live his life to the fullest, he should take responsibility for making sure that your needs are taken care of as well.

If reassurances alone aren't enough, suggest that he treat you to some luxury that would boost your own self-esteem. Perhaps a lovely corsage to compliment your outfit or a trip to the hairdresser for a new look would perk you up. It's the least he can do for someone as understanding as you.

And now, because even in the face of serious challenges it helps to maintain one's sense of humor, here are some lighter-hearted excursions for boys who want to be girls and the people who love them.

## THE THREE BIG HEADACHES OF BEING A TV

### 1. What to Wear, What to Wear?

You've rummaged through your closet and the ink has completely faded from your Victoria's Secret and Frederick's of Hollywood catalogues. Now you're having a transvestite fashion emergency! Well, as long as no one's watching (or perhaps when someone is, in which case it might be even more fun), why not do what all gender women do and experiment with a variety of looks.

Learn to accessorize! Match your purse to your shoes. Match your earrings to your bracelets and necklace. See how a strand of pearls can dress you up and how gaudy rhinestones can slut you down. Drape a scarf around your shoulders for a touch of sophistication or around your waist for that saucy, come-hither look.

Don't limit yourself to dark, drab colors. How often does your office job allow you to wear bright red? Be bold, be free, and be the sexy vamp you want to be. Or, to paraphrase and pervert the old advertising slogan, if you only have one life to live, why not live it as a goddess?

## 2. Will Heavy Makeup Make Me Look Cheap?

Of course! Isn't that part of the fun of it?

Unless you are naturally feminine and barely have facial hair, you will have to wear a heavy foundation to cover up that annoying shadow on your chin and cheeks. If you try to be too minimalist, you will look like what you are: a man in a dress. Instead, try to look like who you dream of being. If you want long eyelashes, buy them. Rosy cheeks come in tubes and compacts. Soft, sensuous, ruby-red lips are for sale at supermarkets and drugstores. If all that stuff is good enough for Dolly Parton, how could it be bad for you?

Again, don't be afraid to experiment. Buy a stack of fashion magazines. All of them run beauty columns filled with tips on every aspect of facial grooming, from tweezing your eyebrows to creating different kissable looks for your lips.

Have fun with yourself. Lock the bathroom door, get into a warm, fragrant bubble bath, and read all those hilariously audacious women's magazines, which will tell you more than you ever wanted to know about being a girly-girl.

And who knows, maybe the "new kissable you" described by some magazine will actually turn out to be *you*.

## 3. Hair and Heels: How High Is Too High?

In my scholarly opinion, you can never get too high.

If you are going to dress the part from toe to scalp, don't stint when it comes to your wig. Big hair goes well on big girls. It can diminish the appearance of football shoulders and hide the mannish curve of a jaw.

An impressive wig (bright blonde, flagrant red, beckoning ebony) will draw a viewer's eyes away from facial traits and towards that lush, feminine mane.

An expensive, high-quality wig can define your look or create a fashion signature. If you invest in a high-quality wig of medium length, you will be able to style it in a variety of ways. No wig stylist will blink if you simply say you're bringing it in for your girlfriend. You can wear it up to accentuate or add to your height; you can wear it curled, to make you look a little younger; or you can go for high glam and have it brushed out full and straight.

Wear your heels as high as you like too, but be aware that no one can step into a pair of stilettos and walk like a human being the first (or even second) time. If you have never worn heels, start small: Even a one- or two-inch heel will take some getting used to. Don't invest in the sexiest, strappiest, slipperiest shoes unless you've got life insurance. The designers will hate me for this, but some of the most expensive couture shoes are the least comfortable. Save the frills as your reward for learning how to do it right. At the beginning, stick with pumps and other styles that support your foot.

As soon as you can walk comfortably in your heels, with a natural gait, buy a pair that is one inch higher and start all over again.

There is nothing sadder, or more comical, than a TV wobbling unsteadily on spike heels—unless it's the time a wobbling cross-dressed friend of mine fell flat on his face in front of a crowd outside an SM club. Fortunately, only his pride was hurt that time.

Practice walking in heels until you acquire the knack. Then let your kinkiness be your guide.

### TIPS ON TEASING A TV

If your man wants to act like a girl, here are some fun ploys that will turn him on.

### 1. Under Where?

To everyone who wants to take the first step in feminizing a man, I have one word to give you.

Panties.

I don't know why this is, and the clinical research is no help here either, but for some reason the very word *panties* whispered into a m–t–f TV's ear can produce a most delicious reaction. A combination shiver, blush, and smile and possibly a stir in his (for now) manly pants.

Imagine, then, the reaction you can expect when you hand him a pair of panties and tell him to model them for you. Here is a clue: The stirring may start soaring.

You have just appealed to three of his most intense drives: his lingerie fetish, his exhibitionism, and his need to know that you love and accept him as he is (the slut). What could be sexier than that?

## 2. The Versatile Brassiere

It may be hard to believe such an innocent little support garment could have so many kinky uses, but a bra is perhaps the most versatile toy one can use to feminize a man.

Of course, you can make him wear it the way the goddess intended. But is it possible those cups might fit over another part of his anatomy? Let's try it!

Depending on the size of the bra, and the size of his manhood, it might fit—awkwardly, I admit—over his precious masculinity. No? Well, you've seen people do it in goofball comedies, so why not try this at home: Have him wear it on his head, with the strap ends tied under his chin and the little lacy cups sticking out on either side of his head. Depending on your point of view, he'll either look like he's wearing a bonnet or like he's a Mouseketeer.

Does this all sound a bit silly? It is silly. But silly isn't always bad, and in the bedroom silly can be very good. Don't hold yourself back having silly fun with the one you love. Turn your sex-time into playtime and give yourself permission to be as creative as you like. Make friends with his lingerie. Sew smiley faces on the tips of the bra's cups.

## 3. Makeup and Kiss

It's always surprised me when I hear from TVs whose wives and female lovers recoil in horror at the idea of them putting on makeup. We live in such a cosmetics-drenched society, and a world where virtually anyone would give up their day job if only Hollywood would call and invite them appear in a movie where they have to wear a box of gunk on their faces to look good in front of cameras.

There are a lot of nature women out there, but there are more women who enjoy experimenting with cosmetics. Many a hapless younger brother or embarrassed mother has been hounded into nonconsensual glamour.

If you like cosmetics and your partner gets a thrill out of them, consider it a shared interest. Here is one man who won't grow pale when he finds out what those designer cosmetics cost. If he does, buy him blusher. Teach him some of your best makeup tricks. Act out your wildest cosmetic fantasies on him. Just don't pluck his eyebrows too fine if he has to defend an important client in the morning.

### 4. Shop Till You Crop

One of the most exciting elements of kinky sex is that you can extend the foreplay almost indefinitely, building the anticipation gradually. Even routine outings can be spiced up with a few provocative threats or a discreetly timed pinch or squeeze. For an extra bit of spice of the transgendered kind, have your partner wear something lacy under his clothes.

If you have ever dragged an unwilling boyfriend to the mall and watched him slowly metamorphose into a giant larva, unable to say anything but "Yes, dear, of course that looks nice," you will find shopping with a TV to be a nearly orgasmic experience.

For reasons that must be plain, most TVs will be very happy to shop for feminine clothes, lingerie, shoes, and all the other fripperies of femininity. You will have not only a willing confidant and an honest critic but also a nice model to hang purses on.

I'm not suggesting you march your man into women's clothing stores and select items for him to try on. But you could. There is no law against it. However, it is best not to alarm the salesclerks with your charming eccentricities. You can shop so discreetly that no one will have the vaguest clue that there is more to your adventure than meets the eye. By the time the two of you get home, however, you will already be well on the way to erotic pleasure.

# CHAPTER TEN

# Power Relationships

## WHAT ARE POWER RELATIONSHIPS?

A power relationship is any BDSM play based on a power dynamic in which one person is the dominant and the other is the submissive.

Many people use the term to refer to a role-based relationship, but I am using it simply to mean a relationship in which the partners agree to exchange power, whether that is for an hour of role-playing or a lifetime of hard-core lifestyle.

Power relationships are not always synonymous with SM, BDSM, and fetishism. There are segments of the SM/fetish communities that like their kink plain: They do not consider themselves to be submissives or slaves, dominants or masters/mistresses. A bottom, for example, may take a whipping from a top for the pleasure that pain gives him or her. The bottom does not give consent so much as permission to the top.

The distinction I'm making here is that *consent* in a kinky context implies that someone is surrendering power, whereas *permission* implies that someone is allowing someone else to do something. Bottoms and tops are, for the most part, hedonists in search of intense physical experience, rather than people who have an erotic craving to surrender power or assert control.

Similarly, not all fetishists are interested in power exchange. Many simply delight in the objects of their desire.

## SHOULD PARENTS IN LIFESTYLE POWER RELATION-SHIPS KEEP THEIR KINKS HIDDEN FROM THEIR KIDS?

In my opinion, *yes.* No child really wants or needs to know what his parents do for sexual pleasure, whether that child is five, fifteen, or fifty.

If you have young kids at home, don't risk exposing them to rough sex games. They can't understand the finer points of terms like "safe," "sane," or "mutually consensual." If they hear screams and run in to see Daddy hitting Mommy (or vice versa), they are going to be terribly frightened, not only for their parent's safety but for their own. Whereas you may be able to predict how an adult will react to such a situation, it is impossible to know what lasting effect it may have on your child. Something that a mature adult can shrug off easily may traumatize a youngster.

Beyond that, you don't really need little Jenny to be sent home from school for doing unto a classmate what she saw Mommy do unto Daddy last night in the dungeon. Not only do children innocently reenact what they've seen at home, but in this case their doing so could result in child welfare agencies removing them from your care. If law enforcement agents discover that a child is routinely exposed to SM at home, you can be sure they will do their best to take that child into state custody. Like it or not, this is how our laws work. The same would apply to parents who carelessly expose their children to pornography. Stupidity is no defense in a court of law.

Some SMers are fortunate enough to have teenagers who indeed are mature enough to handle some amount of information that their parents' relationship is unconventional. Others feel comfortable confiding in their adult children. And some parents just have to sweat it out when they are caught in embarrassing situations.

I cannot cover all the contingencies here. You will have to use your own common sense. But, speaking very generally, coming out to one's children is something that, if it happens at all, is best left until the children are grown.

If full disclosure to your children about your private lives is important to you, what you can do when they are young is to lay the groundwork for a fuller conversation in later years. As you teach them about the birds and the bees, let them know that not all birds and bees are the same.

When they are old enough for conversations about contraception and safe sex, you might want to begin helping them to understand about homosexuality, cross-dressing, and sexual diversity in general. Let them read books about these topics if they are interested so they get reliable information and not biased misinformation from classmates or from adults who condemn sexual diversity. Let your kids know that being sexually different is okay, but do not put them under any pressure to validate your choices.

## IS COMING OUT TO YOUR RELATIVES A GOOD IDEA?

That depends. If you're related to me, go right ahead. But if your parents, grandparents, aunts, uncles, sisters, brothers, and other family members are not open-minded, you risk putting your relationships under serious stress.

If remaining closeted causes you unhappiness (as so commonly occurs among closeted gays and lesbians, whose entire identities must be squelched when they are around their families), then it may be worth the stress. But, practically speaking, there is really only so much your family members need to know about your sex life.

One of the most appalling personal moments for me was some years ago when a talk show host suddenly began to grill me about my sex life. Although I have no qualms about disclosing juicy bits (as you have undoubtedly figured out by now), I was unprepared for his leading questions and his request that we role-play right there on national TV. I'd been promised that we would talk only about my sensational book, not about my sensational perversions.

The icing on the cake was when one of my nephews, a college sophomore at the time, E-mailed me. He'd seen the show. A very sweet kid, he wanted to support me. He wrote, "You never told me you were a dominatrix. We could have talked about it."

Oy! I knew that sooner or later he would become aware of my sexual orientation, or would visit my Web site and see some things that perhaps no nephew should see. But I had hoped it would be later. Much later. Like after I was dead and gone. In any case, whenever it was going to happen, it certainly wasn't my plan for it to happen right then. Even though he was grown up, I felt that the choice to tell him should have been mine and that I should have had the right to tell him in my own way.

Of course, by writing books like these and going on talk shows, this is a risk I knowingly take. I am able to take this risk because my family and close friends know my story and support my choices. In other words, I'm blessed to be able to be myself and still be accepted by the people who matter most to me.

If you feel secure that your family relationships are so close and strong that you will be accepted, then I encourage you to let relatives learn more about your world. But if you have reason to believe that they would get very upset, making a show of your kinky sexuality is unnecessary. Just as you probably wouldn't tell your parents when you've had great oral sex, or chat with Uncle Bob and Aunt Sue about the X-rated video you rented last night, your SM sex life is really no one's business but your own.

Lifestylers may find that it's impossible completely to conceal their relationships from adult relatives. If they spend a lot of time in your house or in your company, the power dynamic will eventually become clear. I would suggest you develop a strategy from the outset and stick to it, without apologies.

For example, you might simply want to act innocent when they ask nosy questions. "Those hooks in the walls? Oh, yes, we installed them to hang plants but changed our minds! We just keep forgetting to take them out."

Or you could take the psychoanalytical approach: "I find it very interesting that you would ask about those hooks. Why do you think those hooks fascinate you?"

Or you could take the revolutionary approach and tell them the truth.

While most of us find it pretty easy not to gab to Mom or Dad about our sex lives, it's different with siblings. A lot of brothers and sisters are accustomed to knowing all the dirt about each other.

Some sibling rivalries endure to the grave. You may have a brother or sister you do not trust with the personal details, or whom you fear would, ahem, get you in trouble with Mom. Obviously, this may not be someone who should be offered a window into your adult sex life.

On the other hand, if you have close relationships with your siblings, they may feel hurt if you don't let them in. Again, you will have to be the judge here, but if you and a brother or sister have been lifelong friends, don't let SM come between you. Sometimes the little hints—a whip sticking out from under the bed, or the fact that you are wearing more leather lately—worry people more than the truth. They might think you are in trouble, instead of having a lot of fun.

Do your best to seek out their support for your choices. Don't announce your sexual preferences to them as a challenge; instead, invite them to learn more about the world of kink by sharing books, answering their questions, letting them sit in on an Internet chat, or bringing them to an educational outreach program that you feel puts your interests in a positive perspective.

Give your family the opportunity to show you that their love for you is unconditional. You will not only be strengthening your bond, but you will be making a contribution, in general, to the cause of sexual enlightenment by spreading the good word that consensual sex between adults, no matter what form it takes, is a legitimate expression of erotic love.

# CHAPTER ELEVEN

# The View from the Top: Sexual Dominants

## THE FICTIONAL DOMINANT VS. THE HUMAN DOMINANT

All-seeing, all-knowing, all-powerful: That is the ideal dominant that submissives fantasize about. Someone who is part magician, part mind reader, part hypnotist, part parent, all sadist, and utterly invincible. But can any dominant live up to this godlike ideal?

While people with dominant/sadistic sexual leanings can turn to Scene resources for information and advice on types of play and techniques, it is difficult to find good public dialogue about what it really means to be a dominant. Perhaps that is one reason why so many people turn to fiction for their role models.

Setting fictional characters as real-world models, unfortunately, can lead to disaster. The sexual sadists in mainstream books and movies are almost invariably sociopaths, criminals, and killers. Sadomasochist erotica, meanwhile, portrays dominants who have no lives outside their roles as sexual tormentors. They exist to fulfill masochists' fantasies. Unlike real-life dominants, no Sir Stephen, Master of Gor, or Mr. Benson has to raise kids, pay bills, or hold down a job.

One seldom sees simple human emotion in SM erotica. Pornography, as a rule, is remarkably devoid of partners who cuddle and kiss or have extended conversations beyond the always eloquent "Aaaahhhh."

Also, while some books explore the minds of the masochistic characters, none probe deeply into the psyches of the dominants. Fictional tops are generally Teflon dominants, people who never get hurt, never feel rejected, never shed tears, and never know joy in life or passionate love for their submissives.

As I said, all the above is fine for one-handed reading. Portraying the dominant as a real human being would interfere with the sexual fantasy that a dominant is omnipotent. However, it's scary to contemplate what kind of damage is being done by dominants who base their relationships on unrealistic models. In the real world, dominance means responsibility and requires compassion.

This chapter offers serious, commonsense discussion about the human dimensions of sexual dominance, including self-identity, relationship issues, and the responsibilities that go along with the role.


## A NOTE TO GAY/LESBIAN READERS

In the femdom section on page 228, I'll briefly talk about the lesbian subculture with the SM community. I kept it brief because, while I have met and played with women over the years, and have occasionally been invited to lesbian events, I don't feel it's fair for me, coming from a heterosexual experience of SM, to try to explore in any depth what it is like to be a lesbian SMer or to advise lesbians on concerns particular only to lesbians. Authors such as Pat Califia and Gayle Rubin have already done important work in this area, and should be considered primary sources. Anything I'd say here could only be a pale imitation of their incisive observations on the lesbian leather experience.

Obviously, I can't write about male domination without saying something about gay leathermen, either. I will keep my comments brief on this too, because—much to my own regret—I am not a gay man.

Gay leathersex has been written about so extensively, thoroughly, thoughtfully, and brilliantly, in dozens of books and thousands of magazine articles by people like Larry Townsend, Joseph Bean, Tony DeBlase, Guy Baldwin, and numerous others, that I honestly feel that a reader in search of information on gay leather culture should turn to those sources.

At the end of chapter 13, page 303, you'll find a nonfiction reading list that includes works by gay and lesbian authors who can answer your questions with infinitely more authority and insight into LesBiGay issues than I would ever claim.

That said, this seems like a good time to mention that the gay leather scene has been the model and foundation for the SM/fetish scene as it is today. In its early days (beginning right after World War II), the gay SM scene was a fairly small, somewhat closed society. Its members, many of them war veterans, used a military model for the dominant/submissive dynamic.

The "Old Guard" of leathersex comprised men who formed clubs with strict social structures, including rituals and etiquette. This earlier leathersex model has been revolutionized in the 1990s as the veterans grew old and faded from the public arena. Little by little, many of their traditions have vanished, and, as some have argued, the Old Guard is now, for all intents and purposes, dead.

Still, many leathermen do try to uphold the old traditions. A "New Guard" has emerged. The Old Guard's influence on them is visible in their dress, attitude, and shared philosophy of respect, honor, and solidarity in the gay SM community of today.

Also, much of the political organization and social history of today's SM scene are the direct result of the efforts of the Old Guard's approach to sadomasochistic sex, which placed a value on love, loyalty, and devotion. Today's gay male activists are powerful and vocal leaders in the pansexual SM/fetish communities.

Finally, while there are some significant distinctions between gay people and hetero ones—the most notable being simply the burden of bigotry and persecution that gays and lesbians must face each day of their lives—people are people, and we all have similar needs, desires, weaknesses, and strengths.

So while some of the writing in this chapter puts dominance in a hetero context, I hope that the ideas and advice will prove useful to gay, lesbian, and bisexual readers who are confronting similar issues in their romantic relationships.

## KEY QUALITIES OF GREAT DOMINANTS

Many people think that all it takes to be a dominant is the ability to mete out punishments and pain or to abide by traditions. The fact is that anyone, including cowards and weaklings, can inflict physical torment on others. The key qualities of great dominance are more spiritual and philosophical. If all dominants worked as hard developing their minds as they do developing their motor skills, there would a lot more happy submissives in the world.

Here are five key qualities that distinguish the great dominants from the wanna-bes.

### 1. Self-Control

Simply put, if you cannot control yourself, you cannot control someone else.

The basic philosophical premise of dominance is that the dominant is the leader in the relationship—physically, sexually, morally, and sometimes spiritually. To put this in very practical terms, think of the punishment dynamics between the master who whips his slave to punish her for disobedience, the strict governess who canes her schoolboy for lying, the daddy who puts his boy over his knee to teach him a lesson, or the dominatrix who forces an adult into diapers as punishment for childish behavior. These are only a handful of the hundreds of roles dominants play out with their partners. Yet all of them operate off the same basic theme: The dominant knows right from wrong and uses corrective measures to train the submissive to understand the difference.

It should be obvious, then, that the dominant has to be in a position where her or his authority is believable. A dominant who cannot control his or her own bad habits, who is weak, spiteful, compulsive, or dysfunctional, is not someone a sub can respect. That's why substance abusers, compulsive gamblers, and people with serious ego problems make terrible dominants.

## 2. Self-Awareness

In order to look into a someone else's heart and mind, a dominant must first know him- or herself. Self-awareness is a lifelong process. It demands an unwavering commitment to honesty, clarity, and emotional courage. It means taking responsibility for one's words and deeds.

Self-aware dominants accept that sooner or later they are bound to make mistakes. When they do, they take responsibility for those mistakes. They do not shift the blame to their subs. It's also inevitable that a submissive will, at some point, do something genuinely hurtful or maddening. Tamper tantrums are a no-no. Self-aware dominants let the sub know of his or her feelings (and may decide on punitive measures) but without viciously striking out in a moment of rage. Sometimes a sub's misbehaviors are cries for help. It's the dominant's job to find out, not to freak out and irrationally overpunish someone.

Self-awareness also implies that a dominant is comfortable with his/her SM sexuality. If you feel guilty about doing SM, or are secretly a submissive masquerading as a dominant because you are ashamed of admitting what you really want, your inner conflicts will trigger emotionally volatile situations that could prove detrimental to your sub.

Of course, even experienced players still have conflicts or doubts at times. More than that, we evolve. Our needs change, as do our comfort levels and perspectives on what it is that we do. That is why self-awareness is an ongoing process. Dominants must continually question their own motives and behaviors and work towards resolving any inner conflicts that could damage partners.

## 3. Sensuality

It may be paradoxical, but understanding how to deliver sensual pleasure to a submissive is an important skill for dominants. Being able to keep your partner balanced on the razor-sharp line between ecstasy and agony is indeed an art. It is all part of being able to manipulate and control your submissive.

SM sensuality does not means vanilla sex. Strategically timed caresses (to their faces, cheeks, chests, hair), the thrilling pressure of your body (or any body part) against your slave's body, a sure knowledge of your sub's hot spots (lips, ears, necks, inner thighs), and long, tender hugs and sexual teasing all fit into a power exchange. The simple placing of your hands on parts of your slave's body will awaken his or her senses by communicating your power over him or her.

The great dominants I've known have all been great huggers and cuddlers. Again, the same kind of yin-yang approach applies: It isn't enough to be able to hit or mentally intimidate a submissive; you have to be capable of making a sub feel cared for and appreciated too. A kind hug does wonders for most people, as do reassurances of love or friendship.

Every so often, you will meet sadists who say that affection and intimacy is not their thing and ruins the power dynamic for them. There are masochists who agree and make good partners for them. However, a no-touchie/no-feelie approach seems to work best in short-term relationships. I have yet to meet any "pure" sadists who have successful long-term ones.

## 4. Competence

Expertise with a range of SM toys and equipment is an important part of a dominant's erotic repertoire. But no matter what the kink or fetish, it is up to each dominant to also learn everything possible about playing safely and dealing with emergencies should they arise. A dominant who does bondage, for example, should not only know how to tie someone up securely, but should have a basic understanding of anatomy and should know how to release the person quickly and safely.

Some years ago, a childhood friend confided that she had just entered into a master/slave relationship. She pulled up the hem of her dress to show me some ugly burns where her lover had pressed a lit cigarette into her thigh. She wanted my opinion and I commented that this seemed extreme for a first encounter between first-timers. She was surprised. I asked if she enjoyed it, and she confessed that she hadn't. She'd gone along with it because she thought this was the sort of thing SMers did all the time and that it was expected of her, as a submissive.

Neither of them had ever even heard of safe words, negotiating a scene, or any of the other basic communications tools that SMers use. As if all this wasn't bad enough, the burns were showing early signs of infection. This "master" had not offered any kind of aftercare. I gritted my teeth and made her promise to apply a topical antibacterial for a few days, and checked in with her to make sure the burns were healing properly.

While this may be an extreme case of cluelessness, I have seen similarly unforgivable stupidity at clubs where novice dominatrices pick up whips and flail people recklessly, not realizing that thumping someone in the kidney area, for example, can result in injury.

Simply put, dominants should know what they are doing before they do anything. There is no excuse for a dominant who recklessly experiments on submissives.

## 5. Compassion

I've placed compassion last, not because it is the least important but because it's the quality I want you most to remember. I can't put this too plainly: Without compassion, there is no dominance. Compassion does not necessarily mean you are in love with your partner, but it does mean that you recognize your partner's humanity; that you know you are dealing with a living, breathing, sensitive human being who is responding to everything you do; and that you make a commitment to care for this person who is granting you the privilege and honor of their erotic surrender.

I will boil "compassion" down to five very basic principles:

1. Don't set your standards so high that your slave cannot meet them.

2. Don't judge too harshly when your submissive fails.

3. Don't punish your slave for being human.

4. Be generous with your forgiveness.

5. Respect your submissive's individuality.

The terms people use to describe themselves and what they do, kink-wise, are subjects of some controversy in the Scene. I've heard arguments from some self-identified sadists and masochists, for example, that "D&S" is not a part of their play, and that using that term ignores important distinctions in the way people play. I respect their wishes to select a precise term for their individual experience of kink and have tried to reflect the diversity of opinion.

Personally, however, I view terms such as "kink," "D&S," "B&D," and "SM" as interchangeable. My label of preference since first getting involved in 1986 has been the simple, no-nonsense clinical one: sadomasochist. For me, it's a kind of political statement. Some vanilla people snicker that I'm "into the kinky stuff," but when I call myself a sadomasochist it elicits a more tentative reaction. I think this is because what they expect of a sadomasochist is a freak, an anomaly, a drooling pervert who lures children into dark alleys. When they meet a person who usually dresses in street clothes, not fetish clothes; who can hold a normal, friendly conversation and not suddenly break into Saint Vitus' dance; someone who actually almost seems like "one of them," then that is the moment when "sado-masochism" seems less like a social disease or psychiatric disorder and more like a sexual orientation that may not be quite as bad as they thought.

Labels are both good and bad. What's bad about them is that they emphasize the differences among kinky people and not the shared experiences. When I see people expend huge amounts of energy splitting hairs over definitions, I wonder if their real goal is to create distinctions between what they do (which they find acceptable) and what others do (which makes them uncomfortable).

In other words, I suspect that if you yourself are at peace with the idea of kinky sex being an acceptable way for consenting adults to express their erotic personae—no matter what the kink involves—then the terms don't matter very much. You understand that all kinky people are in this together, and that there is simply no accounting for tastes, even if these aren't your tastes.

But labels are good too. They are helpful in defining our individual styles of dominance. Labels also let potential partners know, right from the start, what turns us on and what kinds of relationships we're looking for.

So, to help you "type" your own dominant style, here is a basic list of top types, with descriptions of what each term implies.

## Master/Mistress

A master or mistress is commonly assumed to be someone who views SM as a lifestyle, or at least bases relationships on a total power exchange. It also implies that the person enjoys hard-core SM. This generally includes (but isn't limited to) treating the submissive as owned property, giving pain, using punishment to reform behavior, and being the absolute authority in the relationship.

By the way, contrary to popular perception, people aren't born as masters and mistresses. These are titles, not descriptive terms. You become a master or mistress in the context of a consensual power-exchange relationship. In other words, you have to earn the title. You must prove you are competent to take total control—not in your fantasies but in the real world. People who think they were "masters" at age three or present themselves as masters or mistresses before they have owned a slave need some reality adjustment (if not a firm kick in the butt).

## Dominant

Dominants too are the top partners in a power-exchange relationship. But "dominant" is not a title. As such, it is accurate to describe yourself as dominant even before you've picked up a whip. You may not yet be a good dominant, but if you have had the fantasies, and the need to act them out, this is a perfectly acceptable label.

Dominants come in different flavors. Some of them never use pain in their play, focusing instead on psychological control and sensual dominance. They may be dominant in the bedroom but egalitarian in all other areas of their relationship. Or they

The View from the Top: Sexual Dominants 217

could be every bit as hard-core as masters and mistresses, but simply not care for the implications of those terms.

## Top

This label describes people who take the "giver" (rather than "receiver") role in SM/fetish sex. The top is the person who does the bondage, gives the whipping. No power relationship with the bottom is implied. Put another way, all dominants, sadists, and masters or mistresses are tops because they all are the ones who "give" sensation; but not all tops are dominants or sadists or masters/mistresses, because they do not necessarily act as authorities or include pain-play in their repertoires.

For this reason, it's common for submissives occasionally to top their submissive friends in a scene. They can give a friend a complete experience, as long as the friend doesn't need power exchange to have a good time.

## Sadist

Someone who is turned on by giving pain. Again, no power relationship with the partner is implied. Sadists, like tops, don't necessarily commit to taking any responsibility for a partner, beyond the basic responsibility of not unintentionally causing suffering. However, masters, mistresses, and dominants can be described as sadists if they are aroused by pain-play.

## Switch

There is a reason why clinicians joined the prefix "sado" to "masochism": The vast majority of kinky people have fantasies on both sides. At various times in their lives, and for various reasons, dominants/tops/sadists may elect to switch and act out their submissive/bottom fantasies. Some of them switch with their partners, granting a submissive or bottom temporary license to take control. Others prefer to keep the power roles intact and sub to another dominant instead.

This is where terms like "top" and "bottom" become especially helpful. A dominant may have no interest in genuinely giving up control but may find an occasional foray into submissive fantasies to be fun. By offering to "bottom" rather than to "submit," the dominant essentially protects his or her basic identity.

There are also dominants who want real submissive experiences, but only periodically.

One caveat: If a dominant seeks out submissive or bottom experiences more than dominant experiences, then what you have is either a dominant evolving in a new direction or a submissive in denial.


## TRUST: THE KEY TO JOYFUL OBEDIENCE

As you've seen, dominants may play a number of different roles with their submissives. But none of those roles can be real until the dominant and submissive share a bond of trust. When the trust is there, submission comes joyfully and obedience is an act of love, not fear. That is, for most serious dominants, the ideal of romantic SM love.

I hear so frequently from submissives who, after months or years of service, still find it difficult to give up control to their masters and mistresses. Sometimes it is the sub's own demons causing the problem, but just as often it is because the dominant really has not proved him- or herself reliable. Why should it surprise anyone that a dom who hasn't shown evidence of being trustworthy has a submissive who struggles with giving up control?

As with self-awareness, building trust is a process that takes time. One technique I've developed over the years to be sure I'm just as vigilant about the sub's emotional well-being as I am for his physical health is something I call "emotional temperature-taking." I consider it a routine form of emotional aftercare. It's no big production, just a conversation I have with a sub on a fairly regular basis to find out what he is thinking, how he is feeling, and whether we are on the same page. This method has served me very well and perhaps some of my techniques can work for you too.

Personally, I always feel that lighting a few candles, pouring a glass of champagne, and putting some soothing music on the CD player creates a nice atmosphere for intimate conversations. But whenever you choose to talk, make it a pleasant experience. Don't stare mournfully into your sub's eyes as if you're about to announce that you have a tumor. If your sub makes confessions that upset you, don't make things worse by shrieking like a drama queen or otherwise acting as if the world as we know it is about to end. The calmer you are, the calmer your submissive will be and the better the words will flow.

Some submissives will resist your efforts, and this can be discouraging. But someone who is quietly brooding and reluctant to talk is usually the one you need to check on most. Getting the problem out in the open early, before it's mushroomed in the submissive's mind, can forestall bigger problems down the road.

Don't be one of the walking wounded who find out, long after the fact, that their submissives had been secretly unhappy for months. I occasionally hear from dominants who claim they had no idea their submissives were anything less than blissful until that awful day the sub packed his or her bags.

Something is wrong with this picture. A dominant is responsible for keeping the lines of communication open and clear. Unless your submissive turns out to be a pathological liar, you should be able to see a catastrophe in the making.

As the dominant, you should know the submissive's hot points. Is he worried about becoming "too submissive"? Does she feel morally conflicted about kink? Is he prone to depression or mood swings? Is she struggling with giving up control? Gently question your submissive until you gain insight into the anxieties that plague him or her the most, and treat confidences with respect. Never punish someone for confessing their problems, even if you are unhappy with what they tell you. Instead, find it within yourself to reward him or her for having the courage to tell you the truth.

Let submissives know that you are interested in their problems, no matter how small, and that you want to support them.

This doesn't mean you should become a life-support system for a clinging vine. But if your sub had a fight at the office, got a raise, or lost an earring, it's information you should know. If you can console or cheer him up, even better.

General questions are good. I like to start with, "How do you feel?" or "How do you feel about that?" (if we're discussing a fantasy or if I express a strong feeling about something). But sometimes those aren't specific enough to get the sub talking. In that case, I clarify: "How do you feel today? I know you were kind of down last night," or "You seemed to really enjoy our play last night. What did you like best about it?" I also like to ask about work, family matters, and so on, so that I have a complete perspective on what the submissive is dealing with, not just as my sub, but as a complete human being.

Your sub may be so shy that he or she shrugs helplessly, laughs inappropriately, or makes strange grunting noises. Be patient. Don't accept "Nnngghhh" as a final answer; come back to the topic another time (and another time, and another time).

Some subs get so defensive when they are asked to explain how they feel—particularly if they are torn about their identity—that they act out. They may grow emotionally cold or seem indifferent. They may get angry or stomp around the house. They may take their frustration out on you. Their rage may have nothing to do with you and everything to do with their own fears and defense mechanisms against seeming weak or inadequate. Do your best not to take it personally. Something's eating them up. They need your help. Don't abandon them emotionally when they don't respond to you the way you hoped they'd respond. That only confirms most peoples' worst fear: that if they expose too much about themselves, no one will love them.

At the same time, don't allow yourself to be ruled by your submissive's neuroses. Submissives who lie, cheat, withhold information, or blithely break contracts, or who act out irresponsibly when you are trying to hold a serious conversation, may have deeper emotional problems than anyone but a trained counselor should deal with.

But for the most part, emotional temperature-taking is a very positive experience, and one that brings couples closer. Over time, as you repeatedly demonstrate that your sub can talk to you without fear or shame, the bond of trust between you will flourish. So will your sub's joy in serving. An emotionally liberated slave is a happy slave. And a happy slave is one whose service improves and blesses a dominant's life.

## MYTHS THAT NEED TO GO AWAY

In addition to all the myths about dominants that fill popular media and fiction, even within the SM/fetish communities there are numerous myths that some people take as gospel. Below I've listed the top five claims about dominance that find their way into my E-mail in box on a regular basis. They range from harmless misconceptions to dangerous attitudes that can land you in very serious legal trouble.

### Myth One

*All good dominants start on the bottom, by serving a more experienced dominant. That's the only way to learn.*

Many good dominants start out on the bottom, but not all of them do. Nor is bottoming a better or purer way to learn than responsible exploration on one's own or mentorship by another dominant (without serving him or her).

Many dominants have no interest in taking a submissive role, under any circumstances. For them to bottom would mean going against their innate sexual identity. Also, if you are primarily dominant, you are unlikely to experience submission the way a primarily submissive partner experiences it. You may gain a lot of valuable insights, but it won't have the same intense rush for you and you may not go into "subspace" or have any of the powerful emotions that submissives feel.

Bottom line: The only good reason for exploring submission is because you really want to see what it's like.

### Myth Two

*Real dominants don't do dishes.*

One of my all-time favorite Internet spats sprang from a revelation made by a lifestyle couple on a message board. The master casually mentioned he'd just washed some dishes. The hue and cry this set off was amazing. There were those who immediately asserted that if he washed dishes he could not be a real master, because no real master performs menial chores.

The master-in-question, more than a little nettled by this, patiently explained that it was his choice to do the dishes, or any other menial chores, when he felt like it: It was his household, his slave, and his dishes. From then on, people eyed him suspiciously, as if he was a wild-eyed revolutionary trying to bring down the World Order of Dominants whose survival depended on slaves doing the dishes.

That fact is that there are no rules about this. Some dominants believe that subs should handle all menial chores. But I've known a few maledoms who are fabulous cooks, and do not gladly suffer fools, or submissives, in their kitchens. Doing housework does not make anyone less dominant. What makes someone less dominant is not taking responsibility for decisions or leaving submissives confused about what they are supposed to do.

Bottom line: If a division of labor makes sense to your relationship, then feel free to wash all the dishes you like. In fact, when you're done, you can come on over to my house and do some more.

## Myth Three

*A slave contract is a legal document.*

Slavery is illegal in the United States. Period. No exceptions. No matter what you sign or who witnesses it, neither your signature nor someone witnessing it makes a slave contract a legal document. It is not a prenuptial agreement, a marriage license, an employment contract, or any other kind of agreement that our court system will uphold.

A slave contract is a cool idea that Scene people came up with to help couples work out the terms of their relationship in clear-cut language. The purpose of a slave contract is to help partners clearly negotiate the limits and obligations of their relationship on a time-limited basis. It is a very useful communications tool. Couples may find it quite romantic to write one together. But it won't stand up in court. Indeed, if any court should ever believe that you genuinely did hold someone in slavery, you would be liable to arrest.

## Myth Four

*Never hesitate to tell your doctor or psychiatrist that you're actively involved in SM. As long as it's a consensual relationship, being honest can't get you into trouble.*

*Do not lie,* but hesitate for a moment.

In the eyes of the law, injuries resulting from SM are on a par with injuries from battery or assault. Although few doctors or psychiatrists do so, medical professionals are legally required to report all suspicious injuries.

You may be lucky and find a personal physician who either takes a sympathetic attitude towards kinky people or who is at least willing to close his or her eyes to the cause and concentrate uniquely on curing the result. But if you don't know whether this person is "kink-aware," use caution.

The bottom line: If for any reason something goes wrong, be discreet when speaking to doctors you don't know. Use your judgment, as a medical professional needs all the information he or she can get in order to treat the problem efficiently. However, "So, doc, I put some hot sauce on her butt plug to spice things up, and, whoo-boy, I just never expected an allergic reaction!" is just not something you want to announce when you walk through the door.

## Myth Five

*As long as I have my adult partner's consent, I'm safe from the law, because there are no laws against SM.*

Although there are no specifically anti-SM laws, kinky people (just like gays and lesbians) are at risk under sodomy laws. As of 1998, sodomy was a felony in twelve states and a misdemeanor in nine (although in a few of these places, the laws specifically target homosexuals, not heterosexuals). In some states, sodomy means any "lascivious act." That includes the use of vibrators or other sex toys, as well as oral sex and anal penetration.

The law also does not distinguish between an erotic spanking and criminal battery. It will be up to the judge who hears your case to decide whether or not a consensual spanking you gave your lover was a crime or a good time.

While these laws are seldom enforced, and the cases rarely tried, you don't want to be the one poor bastard who is used to "set an example" in your community. At any given time, there are dozens of people in North America who are tried for what we might consider very acceptable, consensual adult sex. Enforcement may also be politically motivated. Ambitious DAs in conservative areas have been known to be overzealous about prosecuting perverts during election years.

The bottom line: Use your common sense and don't expose yourself or your partners to unnecessary legal risk by carelessly broadcasting your sexual preferences. We live in a society that is sufficiently enlightened to provide a wide range of safe venues for play, and which grants us an extraordinary amount of personal freedom. But don't let that lull you into a false sense of security. Know your local laws and use your discretion. Or else move to San Francisco.

## THREE FLAVORS OF FEMDOMS

There are almost as many different ways of divvying up the wide world of female domination as their are femdoms. Some like to give pain, some don't; some like to dress to fit the role, and others stick with street clothes. However, there are three very clear segments of the overall femdom population: the professional female dominant (prodom or prodomme), the heterosexual non-pro female dominant, and the lesbian non-pro dominant. Here is a basic guide to commonalities and differences among these groups.

## Professional Dominants

(There will be a comprehensive discussion of professional female dominants in the next chapter.)

A prodom is a sex-worker who—depending on your point of view—either renders a valuable service to the SM/fetish Community or is a carpetbagger. Second to female submissives, prodoms are the most visible female contingent in the Scene. You are more likely to meet a prodom than a non-pro dom when you attend SM clubs and events. Because of this, people often believe they are one and the same.

Popular media encourage this notion. The femdoms you see on TV talk shows or profiled in magazines are, almost without exception, sex-workers. Unfortunately, using prodoms to represent the points of view of all femdoms is like using prostitutes to represent the points of view of all women.

The Internet has added to the confusion. Most sites about female domination are operated by or for prodoms who have the financial wherewithal (and often the volunteer labor of eager subs) to create wonderfully creative venues to promote their businesses.

I received a letter once from a young woman who, having avidly surfed the Web for information on female domination, had concluded that all femdoms were professionals. Although she had never ventured off the Web for her SM titillation, she asked me to tell her how to set up shop as a prodom. I didn't. The scary part is that she probably found someone who did.

Professional and nonprofessional dominants have much in common, but their differences too are numerous.

For example, of the scores of prodoms I've talked to over the years, most initially started doing it because the pay looked good and the work seemed easy. That's a good reason to pursue a career but it is not the same as being motivated by an innate sexual urge for domination.

Only a small percentage of the prodoms I've known had significant experience as non-pro femdoms before taking it up as a profession. They usually learned their skills on the job, after apprenticeship to a more experienced prodom.

Prodoms screen their clients, but they can't be too choosy. If the client seems mentally stable, doesn't ask for an illegal act, and has the money to pay her rates, he is accepted. Non-pros can be as choosy about partners as they like.

Pros tailor sessions to the clients' requirements. Non-pros take their partners' needs into consideration, but they run their SM relationships according to their own preferences.

Hundreds of different clients may drift through a prodom's dungeons in any given year. Even the most energetic non-pros are unlikely to have so much diversity in their SM play.

Because their encounters tend to be limited and episodic, prodoms don't generally develop sexually or emotionally intimate relationships with clients. Although it is not unknown for a prodom to fall in love with a client, it is not that common either. Prodoms are businesspeople. They have to protect their financial interests. Both money and time constraints complicate things: Some prodoms insist on being paid for every minute they spend with a sub (which means dinner dates involve a built-in premium for her time). It goes without saying that these issues can and do raise trust issues and can dampen the romantic potential.

Finally, there remains a mild stigma around prodoms because of the taint of money. There are malesubs who view prodoms as high-class prostitutes—great for a brief encounter, but not someone they could bring home to Mom. There are also malesubs who feel that paying for SM immediately dilutes its reality, and that the prodom is only in it for the money.

In fact, many prodoms are sincere players; some come into the Scene first and then choose to do it for pay later. More than a few are highly respected political activists and leaders who live the lifestyle in their private lives. And while intimate relationships are more challenging for them because of the nature of their work, this does not in any way imply that they are, as a group, unable to form close attachments. Indeed, there are any number of happily married prodoms out there.

## Non-Pro Heterosexual Femdoms

Non-pro heterosexual femdoms are the smallest minority in the Scene. Naturally, the common wisdom is that this is because there are so few women who are sexually dominant for purely erotic and psychological reasons (as opposed to financial gain). But common sense, personal experience, anecdotal information, and an incredible amount of E-mail suggests to me that a small public presence does not mean women are less likely to have dominant fantasies than men.

There are no broad, sweeping generalizations that can be made about non-pro femdoms, except to say that they come from all walks of life, all economic classes and religions, and for the most part operate fairly independently of one another.

Unlike prodoms (who are visible and tend to network actively, if only to keep an eye on the competition) and lesbian doms (who are highly visible in their world), the non-pro het is often closeted, frequently conservative, and does SM only in the context of a monogamous relationship.

A submissive friend, for example, told me of a woman he served for several years. She was a well-placed executive at a Fortune 500 company. Because of professional concerns, she would never go to an SM club. She didn't have to. She had a bondage rig hanging from her bedroom ceiling that, from the sound of it, would have put the equipment at most SM clubs to shame.

## Non-Pro Lesbian Doms

Although few lesbian SMers (known also as leatherwomen or leatherdykes) regularly show up at heterosexual and pansexual events, there is a large, politically active, and vibrant lesbian community within the greater Scene. Leatherwomen tend to be somewhat separatist, often preferring women-only (or primarily female) parties and events. They have their own traditions, roles, and styles of dress (for example, it's typical to see leatherwomen present as masculine). Their preferred types of sex-play are different too. Acts that remain fairly exotic in hetero settings—such as play-piercings and vaginal fisting—are customary among leatherwomen.

As is true of every SM setting, there are always more submissives than dominants in the room, whether the crowd is lesbian, gay, hetero, or pansexual. However, having attended a few leatherdyke parties over the years, I know that in their own world, non-pro lesbian doms are quite visible. They are not a tiny minority by any means.

What do all the above distinctions suggest? To me, they suggest two things.

First, that when women can find an angle that justifies being sexually dominant, they jump at the chance, and no angle is more seductive than the money angle. Still, money alone cannot account for why thousands of women choose professional domination as a career.

Sincere or insincere, financially motivated or not, these are women who feel no qualms about giving orders, humiliating men and treating them as inferiors, and otherwise crushing them under their boots. Of course, most women are accustomed to doing that to their men at one point or another. They just don't think it's nice to do it to them in bed.

Second, because there seem to be so many more non-pro lesbian doms as a proportion of the leatherdyke scene than there are non-pro het femdoms in the het scene, it suggests that women who have already dealt with shame and guilt issues are more comfortable with domination. By virtue of being lesbian, they have already survived sexual identity crises, and have already grappled with institutionalized prejudices.

Heterosexual femdoms, however, do not usually grow up feeling isolated or judged because of their sexual preferences. They fit more easily into the mainstream because the mainstream is heterosexual. All they need to do to "pass" as vanilla is talk about their boyfriends or go on dates. Their friends, coworkers, and family members may never find out that their boyfriends are also their slaves, and that their dates usually end up in bondage.

This ability to meld into the mainstream is both helpful and harmful. Obviously, it is very helpful in terms of career advancement and family relationships. But it is harmful because it also means that femdoms can hide not only from others, but from themselves. After all, if you lie to other people long enough, you risk believing the lies yourself.

## FEMALE DOMINANCE: OXYMORON OR REDUNDANCY?

Just as women have proven themselves capable of running businesses and nations, they are competent to assume a leadership role in the bedroom. What prevents most women from ever doing so is the internalized belief, handed down from their parents, their teachers, and society at large, that it is unnatural for women to take a dominant role with men.

Women are generally assumed to want sex less often, and for shorter periods, than men. Women are still viewed as vessels, and vessels don't run after the water, if you know what I mean. Women are under continual pressure to remain "nice girls" until the day they become old ladies. Women who wear leather miniskirts, spiked heels, and dark makeup (or who dress in masculine clothes) are generally judged as bad seeds. Meanwhile, men whose jeans are so tight you can almost see the circumcision scar are . . . damned cute, come to think of it.

The traditional model of femininity is so vastly out of step with the scientific research on sexuality that it would be laughable if there were not so many people who still believed the notion that women are the weaker sex.

So let me set you straight. There is no scientific proof that women are less likely than men to be dominant. Zero, zip. There are tons of theories, of course, and not surprisingly all of them support the basic Judeo-Christian platform that men were chosen by God to rule the roost.

For the past hundred years, the study of female sexuality has relied on a model of woman as a kind of monolithic wimp and watered-down version of man. This prejudice arises from religious convictions that women are lesser beings and that, therefore, their sexuality must be inferior to the man's—in its imaginative scope, its appetites, and the ways it expresses itself.

As I mentioned in chapter 7 on fetishism, women are assumed to have far fewer and less diverse sexual fantasies than men. Meanwhile, fallacies about female sexuality are routinely passed off as scientific facts to support religious and social prejudices. For example, how many times have you heard the "fact" that men are naturally more aggressive than women because they have testosterone pumping through their systems?

The truth is that medical research has never proven that there is correlation between the naturally occuring testosterone levels in healthy men and male aggression. (Exceptions do occur in men with abnormally high levels stemming either from a chemical imbalance in the brain or abuse of anabolic steroids. Testosterone-poisoned men may indeed become violent.)

On the other hand, as any healthy woman who's had PMS already knows, the normal periodic rise in our bodies' estrogen levels can turn sweethearts into wild-eyed she-devils. In a controversial ruling in England some years ago, PMS was successfully used as a defense in a murder case. The court concluded, on the basis of expert medical testimony, that the high level of estrogen produced at menses can cause a woman to go temporarily insane.

The men in my life can vouch for that.

The bottom line: Despite a century of medical research into this question, the best theory about why women appear to be less sexually aggressive than men is that it's a matter of nurturing and social conditioning, and not biological disposition.


## HOW TO PUNISH A MASOCHIST

I regularly hear from dominants—both male and female—who have questions about punishment and its place in a power-exchange relationship. Here is a roundup of the most common questions.

### How Do You Punish a Masochist?

It does seem like a poser: Whipping someone who is aroused by pain rewards their misbehavior.

Where many dominants go wrong is in trying to punish a masochist in the ways he or she expects. If the masochist knows a kind of behavior will result in a form of punishment he enjoys, chances are he will repeat that behavior again and again.

There are numerous solutions to this problem. In lieu of a physical punishment, some doms will deny the submissive privileges. Others use psychological punishment (such as withdrawing affection or banishing the person for a period of time). The problem with this approach is that it can seriously backfire on the dominant. It may create hurts and insecurities that trigger bigger problems down the road.

My personal favorite is to give a masochist a type of punishment he or she finds desperately boring. For example, instead of giving him a whipping, you might instead hand him a toothbrush, a bucket of cleanser, and instructions to scrub all the tiles in your bathroom to sparkling radiance.

You can save the whipping as a reward.

## When Is Punishment "Okay"?

Punishment is appropriate when a submissive breaches an agreement or promise to you. Dominance and submission is a contract between dominant and submissive that each will faithfully fulfill the roles they agree to. So if your submissive has given you consent to be in control, and then gets squeamish about or resistant to orders, the disobedience must be addressed.

Before taking action, however, discuss the misbehavior with your sub. Find out if there is an underlying external cause, such as stress at work, a fight with a parent, illness, or anything else, before you decide on what kind of punishment, if any, to inflict.

## Is Punishment Necessary?

It is necessary in power relationships, for a number of reasons.

First, in theory, from the moment someone gives you clear, informed consent, the D&S dynamic should move along smoothly. The sub should always be delightfully obedient and the two of you should live happily ever after in perfect harmony. In reality, people are moody and ambivalent; they say and do dumb or thoughtless things, and even hard-core submissives don't always behave submissively.

There are a lot of different reasons why submissives do things that they know will lead to punishment. Sometimes it's because they feel they aren't getting enough control from the dominants. They may not have the courage to admit it out loud (or even to themselves). Instead, they may unthinkingly do something obnoxious to provoke you into punishing them and thus giving them the control they crave.

Submissives also test dominants. They may manipulate or attempt to seize control. This behavior often says more about the submissive than the dominant, and what it says is that the submissive is having difficulty giving up power. Your submissive may be so accustomed to getting his way, or has built up so high a protective wall around himself, that he needs frequent reassurance that you are a real and credible authority.

Acting out or manipulating and testing the dominant may be lousy ways for subs to ask for more control, but they are so common that you might as well be prepared should they arise. And, if you want to have a real power dynamic, you must be willing to stand the test and assert your dominance in clear terms. Should you fail to deliver a punishment in response to misbehavior, the behavior will grow worse and your submissive will begin seriously to doubt your authority.

## Are There Good Punishments and Bad Punishments?

Of course.

A good punishment is one that resolves the discordance. Submissives are never happy when they misbehave. After all, submissives are fundamentally motivated by a desire to serve and please. Punishing them for infractions, making them suffer for their mistakes, and then (equally important!) ending with a big hug of forgiveness completes the SM drama. Put more simplistically: They know they were bad, they know they had to pay the price, but, in the end, they know the dominant still loves them.

A bad punishment is one that aggravates existing problems by leaving submissives just as unhappy as they were when they misbehaved. Instead of resolution, they will feel even more ambivalent and confused—and, even worse, they may now also feel resentful towards you or guilty and worthless for having created the problem in the first place.

I cannot tell you, of course, what type of punishment will be good for your submissive. It's up to each dominant to learn enough about the submissive to develop, over time, a consistent and effective punishment system. It will clarify the rules to the submissive and, if you add a generous dose of forgiveness and reconciliation at the end, it will bring him or her psychic relief.

## IT'S THE PERKS, DARLING!: FIVE COOL THINGS ABOUT BEING A BITCH FOR FEMALE DOMINANTS

### 1. Wardrobe

Could anything in the world be sexier than the outfits designed with today's fashion-conscious dominatrix in mind? Think of the clothes! The accessories! The *shoes!* Oh my! Stilettos! Thigh-high boots! Bustiers! Lacy lingerie! Leather miniskirts! Latex dresses! All of it in slimming black, and all of it enough to make a sub's tongue hang to his toes (when it isn't busy licking your fetish shoes). Need I say more?

### 2. Slavish Devotion

Maybe it's just me, but there is something about a person who wants nothing more out of life than to devote himself entirely to my needs that really sort of brightens up the day.

### 3. Shopping

Did your ex transform into a stony pillar of sullen resentment at the mall, wandering away at every opportunity, vanishing altogether when you went to try on clothes, and generally acting like going shopping with you was the worst possible torture known to humanity?

Well, guess what: Submissives love to be tortured! (And most of them enjoy accompanying their dominants on errands too.) Just explain that you are treating your sub to a little "mall masochism" and see his face light up. If it doesn't, spank him and then take him shopping. At least something will be glowing.

### 4. Manicures, Pedicures, Massages, Oh My!

When I was a little girl, I was purely delighted by the scene in *The Wizard of Oz* where the Cowardly Lion, after entering Emerald City, gets swept off to a spa to receive a full beauty treatment, surrounded by attentive, doting cosmeticians. It really looked like a good time to me.

As a grown woman, I was similarly delighted to realize that submissives often felt honored to be attentive, doting cosmeticians. Put another way: Nothing beats a home pedicure, especially when your whip is at your side.

### 5. Oral Sex

I guess you think that by placing this one last I'm exposing my own preferences. No, no, dear: It's simply that one doesn't think of a mandatory requirement as a perk.

A *Cosmo* survey I conducted some years ago revealed that women felt they didn't get enough oral sex from their partners (the poor vanilla things!). Well, here is some good news for perverts. Being a femdom means you never have to go wanting on this or any other erotic front. You can have as much sex as you want, any way and any time you want it, simply by ordering it.

Trust me: This is one order that all subs will obey.

### THE FIVE WORST THINGS ABOUT BEING A HETEROSEXUAL MALE DOMINANT

As bad as the myths are about femdoms being man-hating, coldhearted shrews, male dominants live with insulting comparisons to criminals, killers, and domestic abusers. I asked my husband, Will, for the male point of view on the five worst things about being a male dominant. Here are his picks, followed by my explanations.

## 1. Male Domination Is Horribly Politically Incorrect

In our terribly politically correct world, hetero maledoms are painted with the same broad brush as people who abuse and exploit women. Male dominants often find themselves defending or apologizing for their choices. They are often treated as if they don't know the difference between consensual SM and abuse, even though they know the difference much better than people who've never had to sit down and think it all through.

## 2. Clueless Wanna-bes Poison the Well

As kinkiness has risen to public consciousness, and even become somewhat trendy, more and more non-kinky heterosexual men have flooded into the Scene on the naive assumption that submissive women are eager and ready to obey the commands of the first man they meet.

Wanna-bes often think that all they need to do is to say they are dominant and submissive women will have sex with them. And not just any sex, but the kind of sex they were unable to convince girlfriends or wives to give them, which is usually oral sex.

The damage done by this wave of clueless gentlemen has created very real and serious problems in the Scene as clueless submissive women unquestioningly believe that they will be taken care of, respected, and satisfied, both emotionally and sexually. Many find out, too late, that the promises were false and that their so-called dominants are only seeking the thrills of kinky sex without any of its commitments or responsibilities.

## 3. Female Submissives Need a Lot of Attention

When I first asked Will to list his top five picks for the biggest problems facing hetero maledoms in our culture, he spelled out,

"W-O-M-E-N." When pressed for further details, he drily commented, "They're damned moody."

I can't imagine what the dear boy is talking about.

But I suspect he means that women are wondrously unpredictable individuals, filled with complex emotions, ripe with mysterious passions, diaphanous and lovely as butterflies, yet somehow still capable of swooping down on you like a bat out of hell and sucking the brains out of your head.

## 4. Undoing the Damage Done by Others

At the moment, it seems that the greatest threat to femsubs comes from the wanna-bes mentioned above. These are guys who are simply thrilled to have a sex slave, and shower her with compliments and affection until that dreadful day when they realize that being dominant isn't just about getting a woman to do what you want in bed. It involves responsibility too. One sniff of the reality and wanna-bes tend either to run or to hide.

There is also some percentage (as yet unquantified) of submissives who were raised in dysfunctional homes. Even before they got involved in SM, they may have tended to be most attracted to people who are as domineering or critical as their parents. In the absence of clear, consensual power exchanges, these relationships often failed and sometimes failed tragically, torn apart by power struggles and sometimes abuse.

The better part of a maledom's job, at least in the early years, may involve helping a submissive recover from past traumas by teaching her that she is now in a loving, consensual relationship with someone who will only hurt her in the ways she craves to be hurt.

## 5. Always Being on Tenterhooks

Because of the social prejudice against men who take an explicitly dominant role with women, and because an injured sub will look for signs of abuse or exploitation in every behavior, maledoms may become extremely self-conscious about everything they say and do with their subs. The pressure on maledoms to be perfect—lest they slip and somehow be revealed as moral monsters—often inhibits them from taking risks and can make sexual spontaneity an emotionally loaded proposition.

## PSYCHOLOGICAL DOMINANCE

*My husband/master is an expert with whips. At clubs, people compliment him on his techniques. My problem, though, is that when he whips me, I resist going into subspace. He has to whip me for fifteen or twenty minutes before I even begin to feel any psychological effects. Master says the problem is that I am not submissive enough. He says that if I were a true slave, I would feel submissive as soon as he started whipping me. Can you give me ideas on how I can be a better submissive?*

One of the most frequent complaints I hear from submissives is that while their dominants are expert with equipment, they are less than expert at putting their subs "in the mood."

As I stated earlier, if people spent as much time working on the emotional and psychological skills involved in dominance as they do on their bondage or beating techniques, the SM world would be a happier place. I'm not suggesting that doms play roles or act in ways that feel artificical. But learning how to climb inside the submissive's mind, so that you know what the sub may be feeling and so you can play off those feelings, is all part of making a power dynamic feel real.

But before going any further, let me dispel the two terrible assumptions in this letter. First, there is no universal standard on "submissive enough." "Enough" is a subjective judgment. A submissive is "submissive enough" when he or she pleases the dominant. Period. For example, even if a sub never calls her maledom "master," never fetches his food or drink, and gets twice as many massages and foot-rubs from him as she gives him, she is still submissive enough for him if he is pleased with her as a submissive.

That is all that really matters. Case closed.

Second, there is no such thing as a "true submissive," at least not in the sense that someone is born to this or that a submissive's level of submission is fixed in nature. Nothing is fixed in nature; one look at nature tells you that everything is fluid and changeable. A sub who routinely disobeyed one dom's orders might well meet another who so impresses her that he can elicit her unquestioning obedience. The problem is not that a submissive isn't submissive enough; more often, it's that the partners aren't compatible enough.

Now, for pure masochists or bottoms who do not want anything but the sensation, a purely physical experience such as a whipping may be all they need for satisfaction. But for those who require a complete experience of submission, physical acts alone will never be enough. These subs need and want to give you their minds as well as their bodies.

Sometimes it only takes a few words to make a sub enter the right frame of mind. Starting out by reminding a submissive of your respective roles ("Who am I?" "I'm your Master." "You're my slave.") can be exciting for the submissive because it emphasizes the power dynamic. Maintaining the verbal upper hand— whispering sexy threats, saying things you know will make your sub blush, calling her by shameful names or terms that emphasize her vulnerability ("slut," "slavegirl")—will help keep your partner in the right mental frame too.

One type of psychodrama that gives a lot of dominants trouble is the "forced SM" scenario. After all, how can you "force" someone to take a spanking when they just begged you for one? Quite the dominant quandary, no? It is, after all, a tad deflating to "coerce" her into dildo training when the little minx has helpfully brought along her favorite dildo for you to use.

Well, it's a dirty job but dominants have to do it. It is part of a dominant's duty to fulfill at least some of the submissive's fantasies. Again, I'm not suggesting that you become your submissive's submissive by learning simply how to service him or her. But, well, let's face it, your inability or unwillingness to satisfy your sub's sexual needs will eventually translate to intense loneliness—yours.

Your submissive, like you, is in this for pleasure. If you don't provide it, another dominant will. It's that simple.

The key to the coercion scenario is knowing that even though the sub craves a particular act, inhibitions, guilt, or other negative feelings make the sub fantasize about being forced into it. In this

The View from the Top: Sexual Dominants 239

way, the responsibility shifts to the dom: It is the dom who is "forcing" the sub to have this morally appalling yet erotically intoxicating experience.

Subs who need to be "tamed" before they can submit, for example, may be expressing an inner belief that no one could be more powerful than they are—even though they may fantasize obsessively about finding someone who is. Playing the power card, saying things that challenge or defeat the sub's belief that she is as strong or stronger than you, will have a profoundly electrifying effect on her.

Another, more difficult challenge arises when a sub needs or wants a type of scenario the dominant doesn't entirely understand or has never fantasized about.

For example, a femsub may shyly request age-play, or otherwise let you know that she would like to be your "little girl." You may not be able to see the grown woman standing before you in a business suit as a helpless child. You may, for any number of reasons, feel uncomfortable in a daddy role. (Some doms worry that age-play treads dangerously close to incest fantasies or replays secret childhood traumas.)

Whatever you may feel about it emotionally, it is your obligation to listen to your sub's needs, to consider them seriously, and, optimally, to help your sub live out the fantasies in a safe and secure context.

If, after dialogue or experimentation, your see that a particular fantasy is not in the submissive's best interest, it is understandable if you decide to stop doing it. (One hopes you will also give the sub a sensitive explanation of your reasons.) But simply to decide, beforehand, and without evidence of potential harm, that you won't even try a fantasy is not living up to your responsibilities as your sub's caretaker.

I recommend you do your best to reach within yourself, like a method actor, and try to connect with that part of yourself that comes closest to the role your sub needs you to assume. You may discover that although you did not initiate this type of play on your own, it still gives you the feelings of power and control that turn you on during other scenarios.

If you can, try to put your own distinct mark on the fantasy and thus claim it for yourself. For example, "daddy" could still play with his favorite whips, and the conqueror might enjoy tickling his captives. In other words, take ownership of the fantasy by tailoring it to your own needs and desires.

Finally, never get so self-sacrificing that you end up just "doing" the sub. Acting out roles you don't believe in will undermine the reality of the power dynamic and gradually destroy the relationship. Not only will your own libido start to fade, but few things are more upsetting to subs than thinking that their dominants are only doing kinky things to please them. If you simply cannot eroticize your sub's fetishes, you are better off being honest about it. Sometimes you must bite the bullet and face the possibility that you are just not sexually compatible with your submissive, and that you would each do better with other, more simpatico partners.

If you let your partner believe you enjoy it, and he or she learns the truth later on, don't be surprised it your submissive feels utterly betrayed by you.


## SIX EASY WAYS TO RELAX YOUR SUBMISSIVE

### 1. Show Affection

There is no substitute for old-fashioned affection, which is particularly heady when it is mixed with radical sex. Though some dominants seem to think that showing affection somehow makes them look less dominant, my feeling is that if you really believe that the reality of your dominance can be undermined when you act like a normal, loving human being, you are probably insecure in your own dominance and need to work on that issue.

Bottom line: There is a time and place for everything. If your sub is scared or uptight, this is the time and place to demonstrate your compassion.

### 2. Talk to Your Sub

I cannot overstate the importance of verbal foreplay between dom and sub. Words have a tremendous hold over people. Seduce your sub with them. Create pleasurable anticipation by talking softly and calmly about what you are doing or what you plan to do, whisper threats, and paint pictures with words about scenarios that you know will make your sub get excited.

## 3. Rub Your Sub

Massage is a nice, healthy, holistic way to relax your sub. If you're worried this doesn't seem dominant enough, think of it as preparing the main course in your erotic feast. You don't eat a veal cutlet raw, do you? Think how much tastier it is after you've pounded it a little and added some spices.

## 4. Try Tantric Sex

If you are seriously interested in heightening the SM experience to a maximum level, you might wish to learn some techniques of tantric sex, an Asian erotic art. The basic precepts of tantric sex are learning to focus completely on what you are doing. The goal of tantric is to harmoniously awaken (or reawaken) body energies, located in vital centers, by opening the channels (or meridians) that lead to them—use your bare hands, slowly explore your sub's body with gentle touches, and stimulate body energies in unexpected ways.

## 5. Set the Mood

If you have the time and energy, create a D&S ambience in your private play area (whether it's a corner of your bedroom, a dungeon, or the bathroom with the door locked so the kids can't walk in on you). Candles, incense, fresh flowers, and mood music all sensually enhance the atmosphere. Lay out (or display) the toys, fetish objects, and other devices you plan to use, and let your sub see them long before the actual play begins. It will definitely give her something to think about while you verbally tease her.

If you really want to play with the sub's mind, add some toys that you won't be using—especially ones that elicit a nervous blush from the sub—and keep her guessing all night.

## 6. Rub-a-Dub-Dub Your Sub

For true SM romantics, there is nothing quite so tender or intimate as giving your sub a bath.

The very act of bathing a submissive, exploring every nook and cranny, making the submissive assume humiliating positions to expose private areas to your prying fingers, can be extremely kinkily sexy.

You can make it a purely sensual bath. Fill the tub to the rim with pleasantly relaxing hot water and pleasantly scented bubbles or salts. Then teasingly run a slippery bar of soap over her breasts and nipples, between her legs, and other delicious areas.

Or make it a cruel adventure in humiliation and pain. In addition to poking, prying, and putting your sub in humiliating positions, a coarse washcloth or heavy-duty bath brush used on delicate spots will make a masochist feel very well taken care of indeed.


### WHAT'S SO FUNNY ABOUT KINKY SEX?

While kinky sex is a serious enterprise, all too many people seem to think that this means one must be serious all the time. Nothing could be further from the truth.

Perhaps one of the most exhilarating aspects of kinky sex is that it demands imagination and a sense of playfulness. Playfulness is, indeed, built into the SM culture. Why else do we refer to torture devices as toys, call SM sex "play," and describe ourselves as "players"? Not to mention the fact that "play" is the suffix of choice for a wide range of kinks and fetishes, from age-play to foot-play.

Humor can serve a vital role in a power relationship. Playful teasing and jokes will relax your sub. They are a good way to remind your partner that you are a real and decent human being, capable of kindness as much as cruelty. It's also great for downtimes because it helps keep the dynamic very vibrant and real even when you're just lazing around and resting.

It may also deepen the loving bond between partners because it is another form of pleasure you share together and one that can enhance your power exchange. For example, you can tease your partner and she can tease you back—though, of course, she might get spanked for doing so. This, of course, adds to the fun.

Finally, humor is really a sadist's most vicious weapon. Many a sub can withstand a strong arm but will buckle when you make them laugh at things they aren't sure they want to laugh about. Sometimes one sheepish grin is worth a thousand words: You know they really don't want to smile at the cruel taunt you just launched, but they can't help it.

Some of the things we do require total focus and absolute seriousness. This is not in any way to diminish the seriousness and sanctity of SM sex, or to suggest that you're doing it wrong if you prefer solemnity when you're with your partner. But try not to take yourself or your sex life so seriously that you can't laugh and have a good time with the sub you love.

## A FEW TIPS TO SPICE UP YOUR PSYCHODRAMA

The good news about psychodrama is that, unlike overt acts of physical domination, it is something you can do at any time and in any place. Here are some tips on low-risk ways to take your play out of doors without anyone but your partner knowing what is happening.

1. When you go out—whether it's to a restaurant, movie, concert, or elsewhere—make your submissive wear something under his clothes that constantly reminds him of your power relationship. It could be a chastity device, ropes, rubber underwear, a diaper, a piece of jewelry (such as a slave-collar), or anything else he will feel at all times but which will either go unnoticed by passersby or will draw nothing more than an occasional curious glance.

2. Whether or not you do it at home, tell your submissive that when you are away from the house she must ask permission anytime she needs to use a public bathroom. Your sub's squirming blushes when she asks permission in a tiny whisper so no

one else can hear are bound to liven the atmosphere. And if your sub is the naughty type who asks for permission in a loud voice, just lean over and quietly tell her how hard she will be spanked for her friskiness.

That should do the trick.

3. Give your sub a subcultural experience! If there is a prison, catacomb, cave, or other really creepy place in your area that offers public tours, take your sub on a surprise trip. Don't forget to whisper threats when you enter prison cells. If you find yourselves alone in a dank, dimly lit room, a strategically placed pinch (nipples are curiously easy to find in the dark, aren't they?) or a single spank that echoes ominously through the halls will add a certain *joie de vivre* to your adventure.

4. When you get in the car together, buckle your submissive in to her seat belt. Very tightly. Very, very tightly. You can never be too careful about making sure someone is properly restrained. For their own good, of course.

I know SMers who also put their subs in handcuffs or ankle-cuffs when driving. Personally, I am too paranoid about ram-rodding road idiots slamming into us to risk using fetters or metal cuffs while the vehicle is in motion. I'd worry that my sub might not be able to escape or crawl to safety in the event of an emergency. No dominant wants that kind of disaster on his or her conscience.

5. Movies are good. In fact, movies are great. Where else can you sit in total darkness, surrounded by strangers who aren't paying attention to you yet who are close enough to keep your submissive in a constant state of embarrassed anxiety?

Next time you take your honey to a movie, select your seats as far away from others as you can manage. When no one is watching, tweak and pinch your partner here and there, and watch as she tries desperately not to squeal.

If the theater is crowded, use verbal teasing. Lean over every so often and whisper naughty things in your partner's ear.

If you're really depraved (as I hope you really are) and the theater isn't so crowded that you are sitting elbow to elbow, you could also order your sub to discreetly masturbate in the dark and to make herself come while you watch. A nice big box of popcorn, or a jacket or sweater piled on her lap, is usually enough camouflage to keep those around you oblivious to your sadistic little game.

## IT'S THE PERKS, DARLING!: FIVE FUN THINGS ABOUT BEING A BASTARD FOR MALE DOMINANTS

### 1. Blow Jobs

Need I say more? Oh, what the heck, I'll say it anyway. Being dominant means you get what you want in the bedroom. It is your prerogative to set the terms and the schedule.

### 2. It's Your Way or the Highway

While dominance means that you take responsibility for your slave's well-being, it does not mean that you can't insist on getting what you want. Just be clear from the outset about your expectations so that your sub understands what he or she is committing to before granting that consent.

### 3. The Nag Factor

Did an ex ever bitch at you because you left your socks and BVDs in humid piles on the floor? Did your last lover follow you around the house, emptying ashtrays and sniping about your bad habits? Does it make you happy to scratch your ass without worrying you might offend your partner's delicate sensibilities?

Yes, being a dominant means you never have to say you're sorry . . . for having disgusting habits, at least. Think of it. If your sub complains about those musk-laden, two-day-old shorts, why, you can gag her with them.

Is this cool or what?

## 4. Sports Heaven!

Admit it: You may be a sexually twisted, horny dominant, but your idea of a really good time is watching the Superbowl and the World Series—preferably while a silent, invisible servant brings you a steady supply of chips, dips, and cold frosty ones.

Well, guess what? You've arrived! Subs will uncomplainingly serve you and help to ensure that the Big Game remains a sacred ritual. Amen.

## 5. Guilt-Free Self-Indulgent Male Chauvinism

In this caring, sharing age, heterosexual men often feel guilty if they don't help around the house, cook the occasional meal, and otherwise take on responsibilities once believed to belong uniquely to women. (Gay couples, of course, have always known better.) We've all seen enough commercials depicting fumbling fathers cooking microwave meals to know that masculinity is being redefined.

You know where I'm going, don't you?

While some doms opt for a division of labor, you don't have to if you don't want to. As with everything else, just make sure you find a sub who shares your points of view on what makes for a satisfying power dynamic, and you're set. You can come home to a spotless house, eat a meal lovingly prepared with your preferences in mind, and then sit in your easy chair all night, reading a paper. Sort of like Ozzie Nelson with a whip.

So go ahead. Embrace your inner oinker.

# CHAPTER TWELVE

# The View from the Bottom: Sexual Submissives

## THE SUBMISSIVE STIGMA

While dominants are frequently branded as criminal sadists and domestic despots, the submissive's place in the popular imagination is no less insulting. Often confused with abuse victims, sneeringly described as "doormats" and "weaklings," submissive impulses our forebears of both sexes would have found quite normal are now politically incorrect.

The desire to serve and obey—the need to surrender and accept authority from someone else—were once virtues. Indeed, they still are as long as they do not carry the taint of sex. Once "submission" is linked to sex (as opposed to the submission of soldiers to commanders or priests to the pope), people immediately assume the very worst.

To say that this creates serious personal conflicts for submissives is an understatement. To be made a certain way and then to be told that the way you are made is inadequate, sick, or misguided tears down a person's dignity and self-esteem.

I hear constantly from submissive women and men who agonize over whether or not to give in to their needs. Some cite their terror of their sexual identities being exposed—they are afraid they will lose their jobs, their children, and their stature in their communities.

Others fear that their need to submit makes them bad people, or inferior ones. Submissive men in particular struggle painfully with questions about their masculine identity. The desire to submit to a woman goes against the grain of everything they have been taught is respectable masculine behavior. Their sexual needs conflict with the social model for what a man should be.

Female submissives, meanwhile, are often deeply troubled by the moral and political implications of submission. Women who see themselves as feminists may struggle for years to reconcile what appears to be an inner paradox: They believe in social egalitarianism between the sexes but in the bedroom they crave to submit.

Another fear among submissives and those who judge them is that the need to submit sexually is, in itself, unhealthy. The truth is that if something is normal for you, if it brings you pleasure, if it works for you and your partner, and you are both doing it of your own free will, then it is right for you.

Still, some will argue that the desire to submit must be unhealthy because it undoubtedly reflects some early trauma. I won't deny that there are submissives who were victims of abuse in childhood or came from dysfunctional homes. Certainly, those who were traumatized by their abuses face a lot of difficult issues when they explore D&S. Sometimes an SM experience can cause a flashback; sometimes the hurt and pain of the early wound takes center stage in the relationship.

I will note, though, that this is just as likely to happen in non-kinky relationships. All of the non-kinky abuse survivors I've talked to or researched report some sexual dysfunction as adults, involuntary flashbacks to early abuse, and times in their lives when they feel crippled by depression, post-traumatic stress disorder, and other emotional problems that take center stage in their non-kinky lives.

I'll also point out that there are no data to support the theory that submissives are any more or less likely than others to have had a history of abuse or family dysfunction. Indeed, going by the oft-stated contention that 96 percent of all American homes are dysfunctional, if only 4 percent of us come from stable families, how could we ever hope to draw any correlations between submission and abuse?

There is a big negative to being a submissive. It just isn't the one society at large perceives. It's repression.

When a submissive's desires go unfilled in the sexual realm, the need for control, authority, and even cruelty may spill over into their other relationships. Indeed, for some masochists and submissives, the greatest threat to their emotional stability is not living out their submissive fantasies but, indeed, trying to repress or thwart those needs.

A consensual arrangement, with clear terms and explicit agreements, provides both balance and structure and acts as well as a healthy outlet for submissives' innate desires. Without a positive structure, they could end up acting out their basic needs in inappropriate settings. Perhaps the most visible examples in the workplace are the career masochists, people who affiliate so strongly with authority they become the company's most loyal and vigilant servants, willing (sometimes literally) to die for the corporation and certainly willing to put in insane hours at low salary merely out of a need to serve.

Submissive needs may also spill over into non-kinky love relationships and particularly into family relationships. Submissives may take the role of accommodator or enabler, and act out the role of masochist at home—and without, of course, any of the rewards of a consensual erotic relationship.

Again, few people question the martyr-like adult who remains emotionally controlled by his or her parents because, by our cultural standards, it is normal for children to remain indebted to their parents—no matter how unpleasant or downright mean the parents—for their entire lives.

These are just a few of the emotional traps that submissives may fall into if they are unaware of their deeper motivations or unwilling to confront their sexual needs. If submission is at the heart of your sexual identity, it will never go away, no matter how you fight it. In fact, the more you fight it, the more you stand to lose.

Bottom line: Consensual submission is about making a choice. It is not about weakness. Even before you face the enormous tasks of surrendering power to your lover, living out your submissive needs requires that you go against the grain, that you do something unconventional, and that you make a choice for yourself that most people in your position are too terrified ever to make. Indeed, considering the social stigma, making the choice to be submissive demands courage.

## SLAVE, SUBMISSIVE, MASOCHIST, OR BOTTOM?

Just as I offered advice to dominants on "Typing Your Topness" in chapter 11, here is a list of labels for submissives, with descriptions of what each term implies.

### Slave

A person who makes a commitment to serve a lifestyle master or mistress, usually on a permanent basis (though master/slave relationships can be as volatile as any other normal romantic relationship). Slaves grant their partners "ownership" and, within the relationship, are treated as owned property.

Slaves generally give blanket consent to their dominants at the time of their commitment. They generally are able to eroticize most (if not all) aspects of SM that their partners introduce. At the least, they are accepting that their dominants have an unquestionable right to do with them as they wish. For this reason, once they have turned control over to their dominant, lifestyle slaves are unlikely to use safe words or contracts, and often surrender the right to negotiate scenes.

Many slaves refuse to characterize themselves as "bottoms" because of the implication that a bottom is not interested in power exchange. Most slaves are masochists. All slaves are submissive. Power exchange is the slave's *raison d'être*.

### Submissive

A person who submits to the will of a dominant for erotic pleasure.

Although some people use "slave" and "submissive" interchangeably, subs make distinctions. A sub's relationship with the dominant may be more role-play than role-based. Submissives seldom view themselves as owned property but as equal partners who consent to certain types of kinky sex, based on negotiation, contracts, the use of safe words, and other communications tools that imply equal stature between partners (at least before the play begins).

Perhaps the biggest single distinction is that submissives are not always masochists. Their pleasure may come from service and obedience alone. They may choose relationships that offer psychological dominance and control, various types of role-playing, fetishes, and milder forms of bondage or very light, largely symbolic discipline but no real pain.

## Masochist

A masochist is someone who is sexually aroused or otherwise pleased by intense or painful stimulation. The pain may come from physical acts, from mind games, or from combinations of both. Not all masochists are interested in power-exchange relationships. They are best suited to sadists who, like them, are specifically focused on the sensations as a path to eroticism or even spiritual enlightenment.

One of the more famous masochists in the Scene is Fakir Musafar, publisher/founder of *Body Play* magazine. A lifelong masochist and body-modifier, Fakir's radical experiments in intense body stimulation—everything from extreme corset masochism to hanging by flesh hooks pierced through his pectorals—are spiritual journeys into pain. He uses pain for meditation and as a path to awakening.

## Bottom

A bottom is the receiving partner in an SM/fetish dynamic, and is the counterpart to a top. More often than not people identify as bottoms to let potential partners know that they are not seeking a power exchange but either a hedonistic experience or role-play.

## IF I'M A SLAVE, DO I LIVE IN A CAGE?

*All my life I've dreamed of a being a sex slave. I am at an age when I know I have to explore this or I'll regret it for the rest of my life. Can you give me some advice? I have a successful career and depend on my salary to pay various old debts and bills, including mortgage and child support. I have two teenagers who I like to see as often as possible. From what I've read, it sounds like being a slave means that you can never wear clothes, never see your family or friends again, and stuff like that. Is this true? I think I could make a commitment like that one day but right now it would be impossible. Is my dream of being a slave going to have to stay a dream until then?*

When I get E-mail like this, I immediately know that this person has been relying on really bad SM fiction as his source for information about consensual kink. If you read SM porn, you know what I'm talking about. It consists of improbable stories involving unbelievable characters who somehow have the money and leisure, not to mention the libido, to actively engage in SM erotic play every minute of their lives.

So let me settle this here once and for all.

NO!!!!

I'm sure I'll get a letter from someone somewhere swearing that he does indeed occupy a cage twenty-four hours a day (in which case, I will immediately want to know how he managed to get his letter to a post office). But, I'll take a big risk and audaciously state that no, slaves do not remain chained to toilets, live like cattle, or really do anything twenty-four hours a day except breathe.

It is, of course, possible for a slave to be subjected to such strict forms of control for periods of time—an afternoon, even a weekend. But I've yet to meet any lifestyler who could afford (or even wanted) to lead a life that left no room for friends, family, outside interests, hobbies, or careers. We are all human beings with real lives and real-world responsibilities.

A submissive's best bet is to seek out a dominant who knows how to help him or her achieve a workable compromise be-

The View from the Bottom: Sexual Submissives 253

tween the roles required by the external world and the ones you play in your relationship at home.

## ARE YOU BEING ABUSED?

With the growing number of people getting involved in BDSM, many of them for the first time and all too many of them driven by their hormones and fantasies rather than solid information and guidance from reliable sources, it's not surprising that more and more problems are occurring in the SM/fetish Scene.

Chief among them is profound confusion among submissives about where to draw the line between consensual SM and abuse.

The following statement on domestic abuse was issued by the National Leather Association.

### Domestic Violence in the S/M Community*

*Domestic violence is not the same as consensual s/m. Yet, abusive relationships do exist within the leather-s/m community, as with all groups.*

*Unfortunately, due to our sexual orientation, abused persons who are into s/m may suffer additional isolation and may hesitate to turn to available resources for fear of rejection or of giving credence to stereotypes. No group is free of domestic battering; but fear, denial, and lack of knowledge have slowed public response to this serious social problem.*

*Domestic violence is not restricted to one particular group within the s/m community. A person's size, gender, or particular sex role (top-bottom, butch-femme) is irrelevant; anyone can be subject to abuse.*

*Abuse tends to be cyclical in nature and escalates over time. It is a pattern of intentional intimidation for the purpose of dominating, coercing, or isolating another without her or his consent. Because of the intimidation factor, where there is abuse in any part of the relationship, there can be no consent.*

* From the program of the International S/M-Leather-Fetish Celebration. Text provided by Jan Hall. The Celebration specifically authorizes and encourages the reproduction and redistribution of this information.

## Defining the Problem

The following questions can help a person to define the problem, which can have characteristics that are physical, sexual, economic, and psychological.

• Does your partner ever hit, choke, or otherwise physically hurt you outside of a scene?

• Has she or he ever restrained you against your will, locked you in a room, or used a weapon of any kind?

• Are you afraid of your partner?

• Are you confused about when a scene begins and ends? Rape and forced sexual acts are not part of consensual s/m. Battering is not something that can be "agreed" upon; there is an absence of safe words or understandings.

• Has she or he ever violated your limits?

• Do you feel trapped in a specific role as either the top or bottom?

• Does your partner constantly criticize your performance, withhold sex as a means of control, or ridicule you for the limits you set?

• Do you feel obligated to have sex?

• Does your partner use sex to make up after a violent incident?

• Does your partner isolate you from friends, family, or groups?

• Has your partner ever destroyed objects or threatened pets?

• Has your partner abused or threatened your children?

• Does your partner limit access to work or material resources?

• Has he or she ever stolen from you or run up debts?

• Are you or your partner emotionally dependent on one another?

• Does your relationship swing back and forth between a lot of emotional distance and being very close?

• Is your partner constantly criticizing you, humiliating you, and generally undermining your self-esteem?

• Does your partner use scenes to express/cover up anger and frustration?

• Do you feel that you can't discuss with your partner what is bothering you?

No one has the right to abuse you. You are not responsible for the violence. You are not alone; connect with other survivors. There are reasons for staying in abusive relations: fear of (or feelings for) the abuser, and lack of economic or emotional resources. If you stay, help is still available. Find out about shelters, support groups, counselors, antiviolence programs, and crisis lines in your area; ask a friend to help you make these calls. Plan a strategy if you have to leave quickly. Line up friends and family in case of an emergency.

Battering is a crime. Find out about your legal rights and options. You can get the court to order the person to stop hurting you through an Order for Protection or Harassment Restraining Order. You do not need a lawyer.

### We Can Reduce Domestic Violence

Domestic violence does exist in the s/m-leather-fetish community. We can make it clear that we will listen to those who have the courage to speak out. Understand that leaving is difficult. Let the person make his or her own choices.

Keep all information confidential. Encourage survivors to take legal action and seek support. Help find safe housing and legal advocacy. Hold batterers accountable and urge them to seek treatment. Deny that drug or alcohol use can excuse battering. Support changes in that person's behavior.

Leather groups in our community are crucial to reducing domestic violence. Invite knowledgeable speakers; lead discussions; print up a list for members of what resources in your area are s/m-supportive. Educate your local legal and social service system about our lifestyle; encourage their appropriate intervention.

Safe Link is a clearinghouse for materials and questions about domestic violence, specifically for persons who are into leather, s/m, or fetish sexuality. It offers a list of readings and is currently compiling a roster of supportive speakers, shelters, and therapists, and information on understanding and using the law. Call the NLA at (415) 863-2444, or write to:

Safe Link
c/o the Domestic Violence Education Project
National Leather Association
548 Castro Street #444
San Francisco, CA 94114

Remember: If you are unhappy and your dominant refuses to deal with it, brushes off your complaints, and takes a passive attitude towards making a positive change, something is seriously wrong—not with you, but with the dominant. Dominance is no excuse for laziness or mental cruelty. In fact, one surefire way to tell the true dominant from someone who's just getting his or her rocks off at your expense is that person's willingness to work with you to make the relationship as mutually rewarding and joyful as possible.

## PUBLIC ETIQUETTE FOR SUBMISSIVES

This section deals with some basics of slave etiquette. But please note: Although it is written in a decisive voice, it is *not* written in blood.

This is a guide to help submissives gain insight into fairly common rituals and routines in D&S relationships. The etiquette may be a little too stuffy for your dominant's tastes—or not stuffy enough! So use this as a basic working document, or as a negotiation tool with your dominant (particularly if your dominant is either inexperienced or looking for some new ideas).

The basic principle of public service can be summed up in one word: Attentiveness.

Your behavior should reflect your attentiveness to your dominant's needs and desires. Your role is to serve those needs and desires. Is your dominant about to light up a cigarette? Is your dominant's coffee cup empty or has the coffee grown cold? Does he or she need a chair to sit on? Does your dominant have special needs (physical challenges, dietary restrictions)? It is your job to ensure that your dominant's comforts are served by making any and all appropriate arrangements to make the dominant's life easy.

Similarly, it is your joyful task to demonstrate, through your attitude and demeanor, that your dominant's needs always come first. Your ability to devotedly serve your dominant is a standard by which others will judge you *and* your dominant. Not only will your attentiveness please your dominant, but it will impress those you meet both as an indicator of your dominant's power and of your submissiveness. In other words, you will be a submissive who a dominant is proud to be seen with.

Some submissives mistake their ability to take a heavy beating as the ultimate proof of their slavery and devotion. Certainly, it can be a highly erotic type of service to endure heavy pain for your dominant, but what about all those moments when your dominant isn't "doing" you? Are you as good a slave to her (or him) during the quiet moments as you are when your dominant is stimulating you?

Here are some basic rules of etiquette that may help you to convey to your dominant and others that your wish to serve is sincere.

• Always call your dominant by the title of her or his choice (e.g., mistress, master, sir, etc.).

• Never lunge at or thrust your hand out in greeting when meeting a dominant. Wait politely until the dominant greets you.

• Never precede your dominant into a room.

• If your dominant smokes, carry a lighter or matches so you are ready to light your dominant's cigarette or cigar.

• If you're at dinner or a party, make sure that your dominant's beverage glass is always refreshed.

• If your dominant is carrying anything, offer to carry it for him or her (whether it's a coat or an equipment bag).

• When standing beside your dominant, make sure to stand just behind his or her elbow, so that the dominant is slightly in front of you. (Note: Some dominants may require that you kneel in attendance.)

• Do not assume you may take a chair beside your dominant. Wait for your dominant to tell you where to be.

• Avoid starting requests for favors with phrases such as "I want" or "I need" ("I want to go get a drink" or "I need to make a phone call"). Instead, ask for the privilege by starting with: "May I please get a drink?" or "Mistress [Master], may I have permission to make a phone call?"

• If you are in a club or at a party, never bolt away from your dominant's side or give the impression that you would rather be anyplace else but next to your dominant. If something exciting is going on that you are dying to watch, or if you see people you know, first get the dominant's permission.

• No matter how attractive another dominant may be, when you are in the company of your dominant, control yourself and do not flirt or otherwise express untoward interest in someone else.

• Always remember to say "thank you" when the dominant grants you permission to do something. Don't charge off like an animal just released from its cage. It gives others the impression that you couldn't wait to leave your dominant's side.

• Do not argue in public with your dominant. If you are genuinely upset about something that cannot wait until you get home, ask your dominant to discuss it privately and out of earshot of the crowd.

## THE UNCOLLARED SUB

*There is one thing I have always questioned and have gotten no clear answers to: What is accepted behavior for an uncollared, un-owned slave in public? True, I know that this varies from individual to individual, and from scene to scene also.*

*This has been something I have continually been tormented by when in public situations. In public, being unowned, I am always polite. I have no odd ideas of submitting to everyone who will call themselves a dominant, nor do I defer to them. But how would a slave treat a dominant whom she respects and knows, who is not her owner? Some of the things I would like to do, perhaps sidling up at someone's feet when they will allow it, speaks of ownership and service to One Special Person. Calling respected elders in my world by "sir" or "ma'am" makes me feel inside as if I am serving them. That makes me uncomfortable, and to some degree I sometimes long for more, hence the uncomfortable feeling also. But I wonder if I may not seem to them to be disrepectful? I think my respect comes clearly across, outside, but then I do feel odd about asking if they need a drink and sometimes even lighting a cigarette. So, I usually refrain. But then other sincere friends that I have will call them "ma'am" or "sir" and I see how their faces light up . . . but I just can't do that. . . . What should I do?*

This advice is aimed at submissives (experienced or inexperienced) who are unsure about how to behave when attending an SM party or event alone.

Unless you're specifically invited to a club by someone who has discussed doing SM with you there, never assume that you will get an opportunity to play at an event. You may get lucky, but don't count on it, or you'll set yourself up for disappointment.

Usually, people will want to know who you are, or see you around, before they want to engage in physical play. You may, at some clubs, find people whose greatest thrill it is to play with strangers. Be aware that if that's their trip, you will seem old to them soon, so adjust your expectations accordingly.

Rule of thumb: People looking for serious relationships will want to spend time getting to know you first; people just looking for some fun are not good commitment material.

Some basic rules:

## 1. There Is No Scenewide Standard on What to Call People

Some newcomers seem to believe that the SM Scene is so organized a structure that we all know exactly what to call one another (slave, pet, mistress, master). Outsiders, meanwhile, seem to think that we all go around calling each other by our SM classifications all the time.

In fact, no Scenewide rules exist which oblige anyone to refer to another by a title. Most SMers I know refer to one another by first name and reserve the SM titles or pet names for those with whom they are intimately involved.

## 2. When to Use Titles

- Use them when you and your partner(s) or friends have agreed to use them.
- Use them when you join groups that require all its members to identify themselves according to their sexual leanings (slave, mistress, master, etc.). Some Internet chat-rooms insist on such labels.

• *Don't* use them if you are an unowned submissive/slave, unless you know for a certainty that the person you're calling "master" or "mistress" enjoys having you address them that way. Some dominants only wish to be called mistress or master by their own submissives; others prefer different titles (e.g., sir, lord, ma'am, countess).

• *Don't* feel obliged to call anyone "master" or "mistress" if he or she hasn't already earned your trust and respect. If it turns you on to play along, go for it. But you don't have to. Dominants who insist on being called "master" or "mistress" by people who never even heard of them are forcing you into a kind of nonconsensual fantasy role.

Having submissive feelings does not oblige you to behave submissively with people you don't know. Even if you are already in a relationship, the only person you take orders from is the dominant (or dominants) to whom you have explicitly given consent.

If you enjoy calling people by their titles, or if you simply want to respect their wishes for no other reason than to get along, then don't hesitate to adopt their titles and terms. However, if this makes you uneasy, don't do it.

The only one who has the right to give you any orders about anything is a person with whom you have consented to take a submissive role. Indeed, not all dominants will want you to call other people by their titles. They may feel that if you begin calling a lot of different people by those same titles, it dilutes the power of the word when you use it with them. They may prefer the submissive reserve terms like "master" or "mistress" for themselves alone.

The exception: Some online chat-rooms and clubs have "dungeon rules" that specify that you must be in role at all times by addressing all dominants as your superiors.

In these environments, your choices are simple: If you don't like their rules, leave. Don't insult them by trying to argue against the rules that work best for them. There are other rooms and groups that will be a better fit for you.

### 3. Approaching a Dominant at a Public Venue

• Feel free to approach anyone, dominant or submissive, but only when they're relaxing and *not* when they're in the middle of doing SM. As long as they are not otherwise occupied, there is nothing wrong with a friendly greeting. After all, people who come to public spaces are usually very open to making new friends.

• If you see a dominant who seems to be available, or who has been staring your way a bit and you think may be interested in you, it is acceptable for you to approach him or her in a low-key way. *Do not* act as if you are already this person's submissive. For example, do not address them as "mistress" or "master." Instead, respectfully inquire, "May I speak with you?" If the person says yes, then you can ask, "How may I address you?" Let the dominant tell you what form of address she or he prefers.

Personally, I find it very annoying when total strangers call me "mistress." I may be mistress to my partners, but I sure as heck don't want to be mistress to the world! Just thinking about it makes my arm feel sore.

• If you see two people playing, don't assume that the person getting whipped is "owned" by the dominant who is doing the whipping—but don't assume that they are strangers, either. The only way to be sure is by asking.

After their scene is over, you may approach the person who intrigued you. By way of introduction, say something complimentary about the scene you just witnessed. If the person seems interested in continuing the conversation, you may politely ask if they are in a committed relationship with the person they just played with. Even if they are, they may still be interested in you.

The key here is to listen to them: If they tell you plainly that they aren't interested in talking further, mutter something polite and leave.

How else can you tell if they aren't interested? They'll turn their backs on you, ignore you while they talk to other friends, excuse themselves (never follow someone who's ignoring you around a club: that's just creepy), or otherwise give signals that they are uncomfortable talking to you.

• If you already know the dominant, and the dominant knows you, the etiquette gets slightly blurrier. While no one likes a total stranger to begin behaving submissively before anything's even happened (which, in effect, forces them to dom you without their consent), some dominants greatly enjoy when submissive friends honor their power by referring to them as "mistress," "master," or whatever title they've chosen for themselves.

• Do not immediately offer yourself up to a dominant. Do not approach them already naked. Do not immediately say, "I'll do anything you want." The only person who will respond to a clueless slave so desperate for experience that he or she will serve anyone will be similarly desperate and possibly even more clueless than you. That is a scary combination.

• Avoid trite come-ons and forget about the pickup lines that worked in the single clubs of your sordid past. Try to be as honest and direct as you can. Compliments and praise are always a nice way to start. "Forgive me, but I have been watching you for hours and you're the hottest-looking person here" works. So does "May I speak with you?" or "May I serve you in some way?" Speak as respectfully as you can.

• Act with polite reserve, as you would when addressing any authority figure (like a teacher).

On the whole, femsubs can get away with a little more than malesubs, because maledoms tend to be more indulgent about social niceties, particularly when a girl is cute and flirty. Yes, maledoms are often big old softies. (Don't tell them I said so.)

Femdoms, however, tend to prefer well-behaved gentlemen, and may turn to ice when they hear tired pickup lines such as, "Hello, mistress, how may I serve you?"

"How may I serve you?" is very different from "May I serve you?" "How may I serve you?" implies that the sub already is in service to the dom—when, in fact, the dom hasn't even said hello to you yet. If you still don't get it, replace "mistress" with "sweetheart" and "serve you" with "have sex with you" and I think you see the rude presumption of this "Hi, sweetheart, how may I screw you?" approach to human relations.

• If a dominant greets you positively and allows you to stay near her or him, consider it a privilege and demonstrate your gratitude by making yourself useful. Ask if you can buy the dominant a drink. If the dominant continues to respond positively to you, you may even ask if he or she needs a foot-rub or another service. In other words, impress the dominant with your eagerness to serve through your deeds, not just your words. Not only will the dom enjoy it, but you will be getting a delicious little taste of submission yourself.

Finally, remember that high-quality dominants are in demand; they can therefore pick and choose, and the ones they tend to choose are high-quality submissives. A high-quality submissive has self-esteem and self-respect; he or she is not a doormat begging for every stranger's boots. Treat yourself with respect and your dominant will do the same.

## FINDING A RINGMASTER IN A WORLD OF CLOWNS

It can be a sad, sad world out there sometimes for femsubs. Although maledoms are a huge segment of the Scene in terms of percentages, good ones seem to be at least as rare as good femdoms. Even if you manage to avoid the clueless wanna-bes, you may still find that maledoms who supposedly have experience can behave with remarkable insensitivity. In its most extreme form, doms may suffer from "top's disease," a sarcastic term that refers to dominants whose egos are out of control.

It can be very difficult for an inexperienced femsub to distinguish between men who have genuinely earned the right to be a little arrogant or to boast of their extensive experience with kinky sex, and the ones who are just making it up as they go along and exaggerating their skills to seduce submissives.

Remember, it is just as exciting for maledoms to stumble across beautiful submissive you as it is for you to discover that there are deliciously twisted men out there who'd like nothing better than to pinch your nipples and make you squeak. Just as the craving to submit can drive otherwise sane submissives to make foolish choices, so too can the thirst to dominate make otherwise nice men act like boors.

There are other serious issues to consider. For one, there are no good role models out there for het maledoms. Most of them are winging it, hoping to find answers in books or on the Internet, and trying to piece together a solid and moral dominant identity. Some, in an effort to get advice, rely on mentors who themselves are not trustworthy, or join groups whose ethos you simply don't share.

If the dominant has had problems with relationships in the past, or if he has personal demons he hasn't yet dealt with, he may also be bringing baggage into the relationship that can potentially be hurtful to the submissive who depends on him to be stable, wise, and mature at all times.

It's easy to feel sympathy for what maledoms go through. Unfortunately, their missteps and blunders can do tremendous harm to inexperienced femsubs. Complicating matters even more, femsubs tend to have unrealistically high expectations of maledoms. They may expect maledoms to be gods, mind readers, and daddies all rolled into one. What's worse, doms with something to prove will try to live up to such inflated expectations. When they fail to be supermen, as they inevitably do, it can be devastating to their partners.

Perhaps the wisest advice I can offer to femsubs in search of maledoms is simply this: Before you put them on a pedestal, take a good look at them on level ground. Although you may not yet have had much experience with dominants, chances are you've done your share of dating. Use the lessons you've learned from your past romantic relationships and apply them to the men you meet in the Scene. Trust me, if someone is sincere and worthwhile, there will always be time later on for you to treat him as a respected elder, a man worthy of the title "master."

Meanwhile, don't make excuses for maledoms. If they seem rude or cold, distant or emotionally disconnected, don't tell yourself this is "just the way doms are." Doms are not this way. Good doms are, for the most part, nice, caring people.

It may be difficult to resist the shriek of your libido, but sometimes the louder it calls, the less you should listen. Submissive hunger is perhaps one of the most intense and profoundly emotional experiences that subs—male and female—must cope with. You feel that you desperately need the fix, and you are willing often to do almost anything to get it, including going against your common sense and ignoring your gut feelings.

Well, this is a whole book about common sense, so you know where I stand.

Or, as Sergeant Esterhaus always said on *Hill Street Blues,* "Let's be careful out there."

## TEN STUPID THINGS THAT FEMSUBS DO TO SCREW UP THEIR LIVES

1. They discover they're sub on Monday, go looking for a maledom on Tuesday, and have their first experience on Wednesday.

2. They don't bother to learn before doing.

3. They believe everything that dominants tell them.

4. They believe nothing that dominants tell them.

5. They get so hungry for submission, they submit to anyone who wants them.

6. They agree to be an Internet correspondent's slave before meeting him in person.

7. They make a lifetime commitment to someone before spending a significant amount of time with him.

8. They measure a maledom only by his ability to turn them on, and not by any real-world considerations.

9. They lie about themselves to dominants.

10. They ignore the advice in the following section.

## SIGNS THAT THE DOM IS DANGEROUS

Below is a list of warning signs to help you recognize dominants who may be unsafe to play with. It's always possible that a generally safe dominant may, for inexplicable reasons, say similar things to you. But, in most cases, if a dominant says any of the following, run. After each statement, I give you the cold, blunt translation of what it really means.

- "I don't want you to talk to anyone else about me."
*Translation:* I am afraid of what you will find out.
- "You have no right to ask other people for background about me."
*Translation:* You are not entitled to look out for your own safety.
- "If I find out that you talked to others about me, I'll never have anything to do with you again."
*Translation:* I am going to emotionally blackmail you into a relationship with me.
- "You should trust only what I tell you."
*Translation:* I don't want you to think for yourself.
- "Now that you're with me, you don't need to see your old friends or your family. Besides, I don't like any of them."
*Translation:* Your emotional well-being is not important to me. I feel threatened by your relationships.
- "I need to use your credit card for a while" or "I want you to lend me (a substantial sum of) money."
*Translation:* You are an easy mark.
- "You will be my slave whether you want to or not"
*Translation:* I am already letting you know that your consent doesn't matter to me.
- "I won't allow you a safe word because I know I'm trustworthy."
*Translation:* My pride matters more than your feelings of security.
- "I won't use a condom because I know I'm disease-free."
*Translation:* Your health concerns are less important to me than the way my penis feels inside you.
- "A true sub would never do what you just did."
*Translation:* I don't know what the hell I'm talking about. All I know is that if you won't do what I want, I will grind down your self-esteem until you do.
- "You will never find another master as wonderful as me."
*Translation:* I think my fecal matter is odor-free.

- "Everything people say about me is a lie."
  *Translation:* I don't want you to find out the truth.
- "Yes, what they told you about me was true, but I am a totally different person now."
  *Translation:* Last year I was a serial killer. This year I'm only knocking over convenience stores.

Okay, perhaps that last translation was a bit over the top. But, seriously, please listen for such statements and take them to heart when you hear them. Do your best to excuse yourself from the company of such men. Though it may be tough to find a good dominant, they are out there. Set your standards high but keep your expectations realistic. Seek out potential partners who are eager to discuss consent issues with you, who care about what you think and feel, and who view SM as a voyage for two, not an ego trip for one.

## SWEET SERVICES TO PLEASE A DOMINANT

Most submissives get a charge out of service. Service is simply anything you do to help make your dominant's life easier. Some slaves assume responsibility for keeping their dominant's fetish clothes and toys shiny and clean, others give their doms footrubs and manicures, some do household chores and run errands.

Unlike direct SM, performing service is a subtler and more self-sacrificing way for a submissive to show his or her devotion to a dominant. After all, SM play is an interaction, which requires that the dom do something to or for you. Service, on the other hand, is something you do uniquely to or for your dominant, to make his or her life more pleasant or convenient.

Here are some favorite kinds of personal services submissives enjoy.

### Body Service

Body service means that the submissive provides sensual and relaxing stimulation to the dominant. The range of body service is vast. Here are the two basic categories of body service, with advice on how to go about offering them to the dominant

*Oral sex* is by far the most popular body service, for reasons that don't need explaining. Usually, the dominant will initiate oral sex, either by commanding you or by granting it to you as a privilege.

However, you may offer oral sex to your dominant, if you do it respectfully. For example, if you serve a man, you could say (make sure to blush nicely!), "Does Master need his cock sucked?" This is a rather intense little request that will generally get a positive response from a dominant (or at least elicit a spanking, which isn't bad either).

If you serve a woman, you can ask, "Mistress, may I have the privilege of pleasing you with my tongue?" You'll notice a slight difference here in presumption, since, after all, we SMers are still regular people who follow a lot of traditional gender models. So when you approach a man, it is not inappropriate to imply he may "need" a sexual service (since we assume that men "need" to "relieve" sexual tension); when you approach a woman, however, it would be inappropriate (unless she presents herself as sexually voracious) to suggest she "needs" sex. Instead, you aim to let her know that you would consider it a great privilege to perform this delicious task for her.

Not all doms are sticklers for etiquette when it comes to oral sex, and as long as you present your request as a genuine request, which you know the dom is free to deny, and not as a demand or expectation, you are unlikely to offend even the strictest top.

*Grooming* is another type of body service, but is not for everyone. Some male doms are squeamish about having their slaves fuss over them or consider some body services (such as manicures or pedicures) to be too feminine.

Nonetheless, you can try offering some grooming services. These include manicures, pedicures, facials, back-scrubs, towel-drying (after bath or shower), and any other healthful, beneficial body treatments. Some doms even enjoy having their slaves prepare elaborate baths, or will order their slaves to bathe them and brush out their hair, as if they were royalty.

Needless to say, everyone appreciates a good massage. If you really want to impress your dominant, practice massage techniques, either by learning from a book or taking a course.

## Household Services

Some subs love it and some loathe it, but most dominants do appreciate submissives who will do household chores, or take on certain domestic responsibilities.

If you'd like to liven things up and make it more fun for you both, you can discuss obtaining a cute little uniform to play the role of a French maid, butler, or houseboy.

One note: If you make a commitment to clean a floor or vaccum a rug, do the chore to the best of your abilities. In other words, don't try to turn this scene into a punishment scenario for yourself by "accidentally" spilling garbage when you clean or "accidentally" causing a flood in the bathroom.

## IN SEARCH OF HER

I hear all the time from malesubs desperately frustrated by their inability to find femdoms to serve. While I wish to be charitable and extend the benefit of the doubt, I must confess that my experiences suggest that the problem is not necessarily the absence of femdoms; rather, it's the bad assumptions and genuinely bizarre overtures that some malesubs—even experienced ones—make in their pursuit of the elusive bitch of their dreams.

I was at an SM club once, relaxing after a whipping, when a handsome man approached me, stark naked except for a glistening condom poised jauntily atop his admirable penis like a greasy yarmulke.

"So," he said, without introduction, "will you spank me next?"

It was a very large condom. But still . . .

"Tell me something," I asked, "has that line ever worked for you?"

He stared at me blankly. "No."

"And don't you think there's a lesson to be learned from that?" I encouraged him.

The yarmulke bobbled and, poof!, he was gone.

On the Internet, I regularly receive E-mail from hopeful suitors. Very flattering. However, the flattery ends when I take a peek at the images they attach. Almost without exception they have sent me photos of themselves in the buff.

Butt nekkid, in other words.

Now, I can appreciate a good penis as much as the next woman (and probably a bit more), but let me say right now that I don't necessarily want to see them in my E-mail, and particularly not from men who are total strangers to me. Right away, I feel a cognitive dissonance with that penis.

I can't help wondering how many *other* women have been the lucky recipients of this amazing phantom penis. Does the malesub mass-mail his appendage to all the dominant women he can find on the Internet? Is his penis, even now, restlessly traveling to mailboxes in all four corners of the earth, a lonely voyager on an endless journey?

The only thing less thrilling than the naked photo op is a naked photo op in which the malesub is shown serving another dominatrix.

Gentlemen, ask yourselves: How would you feel if an eager woman introduced herself to you by offering a photo of herself romping in the nude with her ex-boyfriend?

Never mind. If you're a malesub, you may already be excited at the mere idea of this.

Seeing a picture of someone serving someone else tells me absolutely nothing about the quality of the sub's service. What it does tell me, though, is that if I should ever dominate him a photo of me might end up some day as part of his petition to serve someone else.

My point is that there are good ways to approach a dominatrix and there are ways that deserve to be wiped off the face of the earth.

If you are sincerely interested in finding a woman you can serve, perhaps as part of a lifestyle relationship, or even something that may lead to marriage and children, then you must treat femdoms the way you would treat other women: with respect and courtesy.

It isn't enough for a malesub just to be there. There is simply too much competition for good dominants. Make a quick assessment of your assets. Ask yourself what qualities you possess—beyond the mere fact that you have submissive fantasies—that a potential partner would find attractive?

Are you great looking? Do you have a great sense of humor? Are you a superior cook? Do you excel at your profession? Are you the proverbial "nice guy," with old-fashioned values? Are you a wonderful friend?

Whatever your qualities, you want the dominant to see them and to know that you bring those qualities to the table.

While looks, obviously, give you an easy advantage, people in the Scene tend to be tolerant and positive about people of all sizes and shapes. Indeed, there are plenty of people in the Scene who care only about the inner qualities in their partners. And quite a few simply don't like "pretty boys" and far prefer someone with average looks.

One note, though: Something that has always baffled me is when I see submissives who are clearly on the prowl for dominants yet make absolutely no effort to dress for submissive success. For goodness' sake, before you go hunting for Mr. or Ms. Right-Dom, shave, brush your teeth, comb your hair, put on fresh underwear (that includes socks), shine your shoes, and wear clean clothes. It really doesn't matter if you're underweight or overweight, if you have buckteeth or a big nose. What's important is making the effort to look your best. What you communicate through your personal hygiene and style of dress is the first impression someone will have of you.

Let me boil it down to one big piece of advice: Please don't wear polyester Bermuda shorts to leather clubs. Okay?

Next, if your qualities are less tangible—intelligence, sense of humor, loyalty, dependability, sincerity, and other qualities that are attractive in a potential submissive partner—then do your best to engage a dominant you like in conversation.

I realize that some of the very finest people are desperately shy in public situations. If this is the case with you, you have two choices: Get over it or select another way to meet people (like the Internet, or a small BDSM educational/outreach group where peer leaders try to put everyone at ease).

There is nothing more depressing than being a wallflower at a club filled with exhibitionists.

## TO SEE OR NOT TO SEE (A PRODOM)

While I naturally wish all my readers to find what they're looking for in a loving, bonded, and romantic relationship, the reality is that professional domination provides an outlet for those of us who are driven by a powerful sexual need we cannot fulfill elsewhere.

Speaking very generally, the prodoms you're likely to meet around the Scene are sincere, well-meaning individuals. But don't be naive. While there are surprisingly few reports of prodoms ripping off or otherwise harming clients, you could be the unlucky statistic who encounters someone unscrupulous.

Before you consider placing your well-being in another person's hands, read the section below. It tackles most of the main questions about professional domination, and will give you a sense of what to expect should you make the choice to visit a pro to help you fulfill your fantasies.

### What Is a Professional Dominant?

A professional dominant is someone who takes the top role in SM/fetish fantasies for a fee. This may sound similar to prostitution but there are some significant differences between an SM sex-worker and a prostitute. For one, SM pros are treated with respect and dignity within their worlds—nothing like the treatment that strippers and prostitutes get from their employers (much less from their clients).

Professionals may also offer counseling on BDSM issues. The counseling may include role-play or may be limited strictly to discussion and peer support. Some also work with couples who want to learn about D&S techniques and training methods.

The vast majority of professional dominants are female. There are male pros too, but they are a relatively small percentage of the pro scene. Another minority are the professional submissives who cater to dominant clients.

Common terms for professional female dominants include professional dominatrices (the singular form of that is "dominatrix"), commercial dominatrices, prodoms, professional mistresses, and psychodramatists. The most common term is "prodoms," and that's how I'll refer to them here.

Prodoms are often self-employed, but pro subs tend to work primarily with dominants or at a "house of domination" (a commercial enterprise that employs several SM sex-workers). This is to ensure that someone is nearby should a client get too rough or refuse to honor the submissive's limits. Some places will employ bouncers to throw clients out should they get too rough or otherwise break house rules. (Needless to say, a professional house of domination is a place where you can expect a strict code of behavior!)

SM pros do not typically come from a sex-industry background. While some prostitutes feel coerced or trapped into their jobs, I've yet to hear of a prodom who feels that way. Instead, they see professional domination as a worthy and respectable profession, and something they freely choose to do. Indeed, many of them have quit very conventional jobs because professional domination offered them the opportunity to profitably combine business with erotic pleasure.

On the whole, prodoms tend to be somewhat older and better educated than other types of sex-workers. The prodom lifestyle is lucrative and also flexible, enabling many prodoms to pursue secondary careers. A few of the top international prodoms, such as Ava Taurel in New York or Annick Foucault (Maitresse Françoise) in Paris, are involved in the arts; numerous other successful prodoms own and operate adult boutiques and bookstores, magazines, clubs, and fetish fashion businesses. There are even a few SM resorts and bed-and-breakfast operations in the United States and abroad that are hosted by prodoms.

Houses of domination may hire fairly glamorous women to attract clients, but be prepared for realer-looking, more down-to-earth people elsewhere. The main standards by which dominatrices are judged are their experience, competence, sincerity, and trustworthiness—looks are, for the most part, considered mere icing on the cake. A gifted dominatrix may continue to work professionally for decades past the age when other sex-industry workers are forced to retire, and can maintain a loyal following of admirers even into old age.

Compared to other sex-workers, prodoms are at relatively low risk for legal harrassment. While prostitution is a crime in forty-nine states, there are no laws that say you can't accept money to make someone lick your boots. This does not mean that aggressive legal agencies will not go after prodoms, but for the most part, pros who pay their taxes, don't do drugs, follow the "safe, sane, consensual" guidelines, and don't cross the line from psychodrama to prostitution are generally left alone.

Finally, it's worth noting that some prodoms do not have kinky sex in their personal lives: If this issue matters to you, make sure to ask if SM is a profession only or a lifestyle as well. If she doesn't know what you mean by that question, you've got your answer right there.

## How Do I Find a Prodom?

Of all media, the Internet is by far the single best resource for people seeking contacts—of any kind—with the world of kinky sex. Prodoms have a significant presence on the Net. Hundreds of them host Web sites to advertise their cruel charms and their numerous fans build sites to support them. Prodoms also participate in Web-rings, E-mail lists, and chat-groups.

Dominatrices also advertise their services in print media. Some restrict themselves to Scene publications, such as the "contact rags" and dominatrix "directories," which are designed to help commercial dominants attract new customers. You can find these publications in adult book stores and at newsstands that carry a wide selection of adult magazines.

If you live in a good-sized city, check the classifieds in your local alternative papers. Some permit prodoms to advertise under "adult entertainment" or let them place ads in the personals section, usually under "variations" or whatever heading the editors created for offbeat relationships.

If you open a big-city Yellow Pages, you can readily locate escort and phone-sex services that advertise domination. This may be convenient to the traveling businessperson; however, be aware that the women employed by escort agencies are usually

The View from the Bottom: Sexual Submissives 275

versatile sex-workers who add kink to their repertoire because they can charge more for the "frills" (and I'm not just talking about the lacy kind). Don't expect escorts to be as knowledge-able as the women you'll encounter in an SM-specific venue. Similarly, some phone-sex operations that claim to be staffed by dominatrices are not. Buyer beware.

Whether you are online or off, the best way to find a reliable pro is through word of mouth and personal Scene contacts. Join kinky clubs, attend educational outreach programs, and avail yourself of the incredible resources on the Net: You will find prodoms or people who know prodoms wherever you go.

### Is There Anything I Can Do to Make Sure a Prodom Is Safe?

Again, I can't overemphasize the importance of word-of-mouth recommendations. It is in your best interest—both psychically and financially— to check on a dominant's background and be sure that he or she has not left a trail of broken hearts or empty wallets behind. (Unless, of course, getting rejected and robbed is your fetish.)

If possible, ask around to see if a prodom you've contacted is known to others. If you don't belong to any groups or have any SM contacts, then you can try leaving a message on UseNet. Most sincere prodoms are involved with the SM Scene in their areas. If a pro cannot give you the name of a single Scene person who can vouch for her (very important: it should be some-one who knows her in real life, not an "E-mail slave" or someone who only knows her online), then move on.

I wish I didn't have to add this next sentence, but I will any-way. If you learn that a dominatrix injured someone or did not stop when the submissive used his safe word, run the other way. Do not give her the benefit of the doubt when your health is at stake.

### What Do I Say When I Contact Her?

Whether you call, E-mail, or talk to her in person, your presession interaction should be meaningful. It isn't enough to flirt or drop hints. At a minimum, you should have at least one serious conversation with the prodom before you let her lay a hand on you. It doesn't necessarily have to be a long talk, but you should make sure that she understands what you want and will respect your limits. Most prodoms are willing to answer a new client's questions, but don't abuse the privilege or waste her time. She is a businesswoman who depends on fees for her services. If you find that you need to speak with her at length, make an appointment for a counseling session with her and pay her for her time.

The most difficult step for most men seeking out prodoms is getting over those shy, awkward first moments on the phone. You will get your first hint about a prodom by the way she handles the conversation. Does she seem friendly, knowledgeable, understanding, and supportive? A good dominatrix should be able to put you at ease and help make the process easy for you. If she comes across as hostile, indifferent, forgetful, or cold, I would recommend you avoid her.

Do not think that just because you contact a dominant you are obliged to use her service. You may contact several before selecting the one who best suits you. Unless you crave variety, your best bet is to find one understanding dominatrix who you like and respect, and then return to her. The longer you remain with a dominant, the better she will understand your quirks and limits, and the better she will be able to satisfy you.

For the most part, prodoms are chatty, savvy, and efficient people who will ask you a lot of questions. Some may even have you fill out a form with detailed questions about your experience and health status. But if they don't, here are the five important areas you need to discuss before playing.

1. *Her Specialties:* Not all prodoms are good at (or enjoy) all fantasy scenarios. Some who are fabulous with a whip have little or no understanding of infantilization, and vice versa. So when you speak with her, ask if she is familiar with your type of fantasies, and whether she's had experience with them.

A fair number of prodoms specialize in particular scenes. If you can find one who has a special fondness for the kink you are interested in, she should make the top of your list. Indeed, finding someone whose kinks are compatible with yours is generally far more important than finding someone who is closer to your ideal physical type.

2. *Your Fantasies:* A prodom is well acquainted with every dark recess of the human sexual imagination. You need not be ashamed to reveal your fantasies to her.

Tell her, in as clear detail as you can muster, what fantasies you wish to act out. This will allow her to prepare accordingly—not just in terms of equipment but also in terms of her mindset. She will most likely plan your time together carefully before you arrive.

If you don't know what you want, figure it out before you call. Or, as I said earlier, schedule an appointment simply to talk. Most prodoms have clients who visit only to talk, so your request won't sound strange.

3. *Her Fees:* Prodom rates vary widely, depending on the location, experience, reputation, and attractiveness of the dominatrix. Top dominatrices in New York and Paris charge hundreds of dollars for a single hour or thousands for a day. In smaller cities, you will usually pay less. Generally speaking, you can expect to pay between $150 and $350 for an hour-long session. (If she has to travel to see you, she will expect you to cover her expenses.)

Prodoms' fees are seldom negotiable. Like all professionals, they expect a certain rate for their services, and expect you to honor their standard. It is possible that a prodom may offer you a break (particularly if you prepay for a few sessions), but don't insult her by haggling over price.

4. *Safe Words and Limits:* A pro should discuss safe words and limits with you before she places a hand on you. If she doesn't, something is fishy, because this basic discussion has become a standard in the industry. Ask her directly if she uses safe words and whether she respects limits. If she doesn't know what you're talking about, or says no to either question, do not make the appointment. If you're already there when you find out, leave.

5. *Your Health Situation:* Although this is a tough topic to talk about, it is critical that you honestly discuss any and all medical conditions you may have. This includes but is not limited to asthma, diabetes, epilepsy, arthritis, Tourette's, impotence, a heart condition, major surgeries, medications you are taking, and any other health issues.

Most responsible dominants will ask about your health. If they don't, make it your business to enlighten them. If a dominant doesn't seem to be paying attention, or does not take your special needs into account, do not use her services. You do not want to go into insulin shock while in bondage or to have an asthma attack with a gag in your mouth. Nor do you want an old back problem to act up while you're kneeling. Even masochists have a hard time eroticizing a bad back.

## What You Should Expect from a Prodom

*Expect . . . Compassion:* Even if you are a heavy masochist who has selected a heavy sadist, you should expect the prodom to be compassionate with you. This means that she expresses concern for your well-being, makes sure that you feel safe, and does not abuse her power over you. More than that, she should demonstrate sensitivity to your particular sexual needs and use good judgment so that your session is a positive experience for you both.

*Expect . . . A Fair Return for Your Money:* When you visit a professional dominant, you are paying for a service. You are entitled to receive what you pay for. This doesn't mean the prodom is yours to boss around (that kind of attitude will probably get you thrown out) or that you can dictate the rules. What it does mean, however, is that by taking your money she contracts to help you fulfill your fantasy to the best of her abilities.

In some cases, submissives come away disappointed because they were not honest about what they really wanted. A prodom cannot control that. If you didn't tell her, don't expect her to read your mind. However, she should demonstrate that she's given thought to your session by wearing the appropriate outfit, having the right toys handy, knowing what kinds of things to say to turn you on, and otherwise tailoring the session to your needs. That is her job.

*Expect . . . A Safe, Secure Environment:* A professional dominatrix should have the accoutrements of her profession. Not only should she have a wardrobe adequate to live out the role you want her to play, but she should have the toys and equipment to enact the fantasy. Her equipment should be sturdy and clean. She should be absolutely, scrupulously AIDS-aware and sterilize her toys after each client. Her place should be neat, clean, and decently furnished. The building should be located in a reasonably safe part of town, and the premises should look and feel secure.

It should also be a drug- and alcohol-free environment. If the dominatrix or her coworkers appear intoxicated, leave immediately.

## What You Should Not Expect

*Don't Expect . . . Sex:* In all states but Nevada, sex-workers can be arrested for prostitution if they remove their clothes for lewd purpose. So don't be surprised if the dominant remains fully clad and refuses any type of sexual contact. Some prodoms may not even allow you to masturbate on their premises.

Though Nevada is the only state where prostitution is legal, you will, from time to time, find prodoms in other states who agree to sex. If you accept, be aware that you are breaking the law with her. While courts are usually tougher on sex-workers than on their clients, I think most people would, on the whole, prefer not to stand in a public courtroom, testifying about the spanking they just paid for.

*Don't Expect . . . Total Compliance:* Although you should expect a fair return for your fee, don't expect a prodom to go along with every single thing that you want. Once you have negotiated your session with her, and described your fantasies, it is time for you to let go and let her do what she is good at.

It's quite possible that she will try things on you that you didn't specifically request, just as she may not deliver every single item on the menu you handed her. After all, she is the dominatrix. She must demonstrate her power and control over you in real ways or she won't be credible in the role.

If what you really want is just any woman who will act out your fantasies exactly as you've scripted them, without any ideas or will of her own, you will likely come away from a real-life visit very disappointed.

*Don't Expect . . . Criminal Activity:* While prodoms will act out most consensual SM/fetish fantasies, don't expect them to fulfill fantasies that are violent or involve people who cannot give informed consent. She may be willing to role-play extreme fantasies with you (in which you or she pretends to be doing something against the law), but no dominant in her right mind will engage in actual rape, incest, pedophilia, necrophilia, or other sex act that is criminal by definition. A prodom must know exactly where to draw the line between fantasy and reality. If she doesn't, she is dangerous to herself, to her community, and especially to you.

As I said earlier, drugs, prostitution, and other blatant criminal activities are also out of the question. A sane dominant would rather lose your business than risk arrest.

*Don't Expect . . . The World According to de Sade:* Contrary to popular opinion, prodoms are not one-dimensional figures straight out of the pages of smutty novels. They are normal people, with family lives and friends, who make a living at something they enjoy—just as you enjoy it.

Their "dungeons" will not, for the most part, look like the medieval dungeons of lore. There should be enough equipment on hand to enact a range of fantasies, but don't be surprised if a prodom who works out of her house leads you through a middle-class home to a back bedroom with only a few pieces of large-scale equipment and a few dozen whips and clips hanging on the walls. If you can't stand a little dose of reality with your fantasy, let the dominant know before you get there and she will try to shield you from the dreadful truth that she is a real human being.

Houses of domination are, on the whole, more "atmospheric," because no one lives there: They have been designed specifically as a kind of kinky fun house. They have more space, and usually more funds, to install all kinds of fancy gizmos. Still, even pro houses will look like what they are—venues for adult entertainment—and not like monasteries in Europe.

# CHAPTER THIRTEEN

# Kinky Facts, Follies, and Fun

All good things must come to an end, even in kinky sex. And so we come to the last chapter of this book. To round things off, I'm ending with a potpourri of advice, games, and information that I hope will enlighten and entertain you and remain a resource for you for years to come. Some of the advice will seem familiar to you, as it restates points I've made throughout the book. For instance, in "Reviewing the Rules," page 284, I stress for one last time ten basic guidelines on kinky sex-play.

I hope that this book has helped broaden your understanding of kinky sex—what it is and what it is not. If this book has opened new possibilities for you or raised new questions in your mind, please take the time to think them through before jumping into anything. The more you understand about the natural diversity of human sexuality and the more aware you become of your own sexual needs, the more erotic pleasure you will glean from life and the stronger your relationships will grow.

You might want to return and retake quizzes such as "Ready . . . or Not?" (page 40) to see whether you score differently. Similarly, if the book has emboldened you to talk to your partner or to begin exploring the world of kink, it's a good time to review the various communication tools and etiquette guidelines in the preceding chapters. Don't hesitate to modify tools or quizzes I've created to better suit the needs of your own relationships.

At the end of this chapter, I'll provide you with an informal bibliography of nonclinical books by and for kinky people to help you continue to learn about these issues. If you have access to the Internet, visit my Kink Links Catalogue (gloria-brame.com/love8.htm). As a free service to kinky people, the

Catalogue offers thousands of links to high-quality Web sites, mailing lists, social organizations, chat-groups, and more.

Use my insights as jumping-off points, not terminal destinations. While I have written the truth as I know it, based upon both my own experiences and all the research I could gather, I did not try to represent all points of view. Instead, I've given you my personal and scholarly understandings of the chief issues kinky people face. I expect some readers to disagree with me. So, debate the issues with trusted friends, bring this book to reading salons and share it with lovers, or start a diary for thoughts and reactions to what's written here.

My goal here has been to open your eyes to the possibilities so you have the information to make the right decisions for yourself. I wanted simply to state the truth as I know it: that sex is not dirty, and that what consenting adults choose to do together in private is no one's business but their own.

Finally, I'd like to wish you bon voyage (and "bon courage") if you embark on the lifelong journey into a full understanding of your sexual identity. As you travel, remember that a kinky relationship is successful when it brings you joy and affirms your value as a human being.

Play safe. Play smart. Keep it consensual.

## REVIEWING THE RULES

For some, BDSM/fetish sex is truly a sacred realm, which carries certain spiritual obligations. For others, it a high-intensity hedonistic sport that must be played with maximum attention to physical safety. Then there are those who see SM/leather as an organized society, rich with tradition, as well as a culture with its own social and political concerns. Others believe that "what it is that we do" or "WIITWD" (as kink is referred to on the Internet) is purely sexual fun, nothing more or less. And some of us believe it's a bit of all of the above.

Because BDSM/fetishism means different things to different people, there is a continual debate within groups and clubs about what we do, why we do it, and how we do it. Sometimes these debates turn into raging controversies, as individuals set forth passionate arguments about everything from safe words and slave contracts to the very meaning of "safe," "sane," and "consensual."

Still, while customs, morals, opinions, and ways of doing SM/fetish sex vary from group to group, and indeed from individual to individual, certain ethical understandings are fairly universal in the Scene. Below, I've tried to articulate the ten most important ones, with explanations of what each one means.

## Ten Rules to Remember

1. *Obtain informed consent.* This is the first and most important moral principle among members of the organized BDSM and fetish communities.

Informed consent means your partner is of legal age to give consent and clearly understands what he or she is agreeing to do with you. Obviously, this rules out sex with underaged individuals or people who are incapable of making good choices for themselves.

If a potential partner does not give consent, your options are either to redirect your energies to a different area of erotic play or to seek out a different partner.

2. *Educate yourself.* Kinky sex is like gardening: The more you know about the hows and whys of it, the more you realize how very little you know. (Actually, it's better than gardening, because you don't dump big bags of manure on your beds. Unless you're *really* kinky.)

Anyway, my point is that kinky sex is not a question of picking up a few bondage and spanking techniques. It's an evolving process, in which every year of your life brings new insights, feelings, and experiences.

Hands-on experience is the best teacher. But in addition to whatever you may learn from your intimate relationships, you owe it to yourself to learn about the forces that drive you. Read as many books as you can, attend seminars and symposia, and find like-minded people who can discuss these subjects with you in a frank, mature, and enlightened way.

3. *Educate your partner.* It isn't enough for you to be educated. Whether you are the dominant or the submissive, introduce your partner to reading and other materials that open the door to new understandings of kinky sex. Read books together, rent videos, and discuss articles or ideas that you find interesting. Keep the lines of communication open by using these materials to discuss your own likes and dislikes, and to reach new levels of mutual understanding as a couple.

4. *Know your limits.* Whether you are dominant, submissive, shades of both, or neither, your first task should be to figure out what turns you on and what turns you off. Although your limits may change over time—or may, when you are involved with someone you deeply trust, be more flexible than you expected—knowing where to draw the line is crucial to playing safely. Of course, everyone has a different line: Some people don't like pain, others don't care for watersports, and still others can't stand the thought of a piercing.

Unfortunately, many of us, thinking we're being nice, will let people talk us into trying things that make us queasy. Don't let anyone else convince you that because they feel okay with something you should be willing to do it to them or for them. I have talked to dozens of people, both dominant and submissive, who reluctantly agreed to act out a partner's fantasies, only to regret it later and end up resenting the person they had indulged.

5. *Respect your partner's limits.* Before you begin playing with someone, it is your obligation (to them and to yourself) to find out what limits they have. This includes any diseases or physical challenges they have that may restrict the types of play they can do.

If they are unsure of their limits, and particularly if they are very new to this, your best bet is to proceed very cautiously. If you're the dominant, it is your job to ensure that you don't accidentally push someone to a point where he or she begins to react badly. If your submissive regularly has significant emotional distress either during or after sex, chances are that you do not fully understand his or her limits.

If you're submissive, do not assume that your dominant wants to take a fantasy as far as you want to go. You may encounter tops or dominants whose tastes are milder than your own. This is a normal incompatibility. Don't try to manipulate them to give you more. If you cannot find satisfaction with a partner because he or she doesn't give you the level of pain you want, then you need to find a new dominant.

6. *Make commitments you can keep.* In the first flush of kinky romance, dominants and submissives often make passionate commitments based on their hormones and not their heads. I've known people who have relocated to other cities and given up jobs, families, and friends to be with their one true love, only to discover, when reality sinks in, that they cannot go through with a full-time master/slave relationship.

Here is some basic, blunt advice. Don't promise to be someone's master if you have never even met the person. Don't lead anyone to believe you are ready to dominate them full-time unless you have had enough experience as a dominant to understand all the responsibilities of the role.

Don't commit to being a slave if you've never tried SM before. Don't make wild promises to a dominant in the heat of passion that you later realize you could never fulfill.

Before you tell someone you are going to either take care of them or serve them, be sure you understand exactly what is involved and know in your heart that this is indeed someone you will be able to live with until the end of your life.

Master/slave relationships are every bit as serious as marriages. Some SMers would say they are, in fact, more so, because of the emotional intensity of the power dynamic. So remember that when you make a commitment, the other person is relying on you to fulfill it.

7. *Know your equipment.* If you are going to use a toy— whether it's something as seemingly harmless as a dildo or as menacing as a heavy whip—you must know everything you can about its uses, its effects, its limits, and its risks. Even the most harmless toy can cause harm if it is used improperly. Similarly, even the most menacing ones can be used so benevolently as to create an entirely sensual experience.

Most people recommend that you gradually get to understand your equipment by experimenting with it—carefully—on yourself first. Dominants will try out a whip by slapping it on their forearm, and judge clamps by attaching them to the web of skin between thumb and forefinger. However you go about it, take time getting to know each new toy.

Nearly all SM/fetish clubs and organizations offer educational outreach programs that include "demos" (demonstrations) on the proper use of different types of equipment. Whether you want to learn about fisting and watersports, or the way to deliver a whipping that will bring your partner to ecstasy, the resources exist for you to learn through observation and discussion. If you can't get to such a club, then go online. You can find tons of valuable information about technique on the Web, and you can ask people for their advice on message boards and in chat-rooms throughout the Internet.

8. *Stay calm.* A lot of things can happen during kinky sex. Some people have flashbacks to childhood traumas or panic attacks that upset them deeply, causing them to cry or feel dizzy. Knots can slip, causing hands or feet to get numb. Backs can give out, making bondage impossible. Mind games, humiliation, and even nakedness can elicit powerful emotional reactions.

Whether you are dominant or submissive, you must always be prepared for the possibility that something you weren't expecting may happen. For some of us, this is part of the thrill. The more passionate and adventurous you are, the more likely this is. But even difficult moments can have happy, exhilarating conclusions if both partners remain clearheaded and work through it together. Still, in the moment, sudden changes may threaten to cause a crisis situation.

It is crucial for both dominant and submissive to be able to remain calm should something go wrong. If you're the dom, speak calmly and confidently, reassuring the sub that you can and will take care of it. If you're the sub, try not to panic: Let the dom do his or her job. If your handcuffs suddenly got tight, it won't help matters if you flop around like a tuna while your dom is trying to unlock them. If your dominant offers you comfort, take it. If your submissive needs your comfort, give it.

Work together, like any two people facing a small, temporary crisis, and get through it with love, cooperating in as patient and mature a fashion as you can.

(I guess Adult Babies are off the hook on this one.)

9. *Expect pleasure.* Why do we do kinky sex? We do it because it brings pleasure to our lives.

Whatever it is you seek from kinky sexy, whether it is an erotic thrill, spiritual fulfillment, or anything else, don't compromise: If you are feeling unhappy or continually frustrated by your interaction with your partner, it's time to sit down and reevaluate the relationship. This applies to dominants as well as to submissives. Even if you have already signed a contract with the person, it may be time to renegotiate it and to suggest improvements.

This doesn't mean that you should abandon a relationship the minute problems arise or run away when life crises temporarily thwart intimacy. If you promised someone you'd stick by him through thick and thin, don't selfishly use the pleasure principle as an easy out. However, if there are fundamental sexual incompatibilities; if your partner cannot or will not work with you towards a happy solution; if you spend more time being unhappy than happy about your relationship—then *it is time to make a change for the positive.*

10. *Love yourself.* I won't issue the usual cliché about how you need to love yourself in order to love others (whoops, I just did—I'm sneaky that way). What I mean by loving yourself here is simply this: You are not a bad person for needing kinky sex. Being kinky does not make you better or worse than anyone else; it does not make you less human, or less capable of kindness, generosity, or clear moral standards.

Your sexual identity is something that was formed early in your life (perhaps even at birth, perhaps even in the womb—science has yet to reveal to us the answers to these mysteries). You had no control over it. What you do control is how you live today.

Love yourself. Respect yourself. And most of all, believe in your value as a human being. Everyone deserves to be loved.

## DATA TO DIGEST

You've seen a number of clinical and scientific data cited throughout the book. The following data, however, comes directly from Scene sources. The New England chapter of the National Leather Association (NLA) drew 2,000 people to its December 1998 Fetish Fair Fleamarket in Boston, and conducted an informal exit survey at the event, polling roughly 200 people.

Participants were given a list of ten issues and asked to rank them in order of importance. The two top concerns listed by those polled were (1) the social stigma associated with being kinky and (2) feeling isolated and unable to find BDSM resources.

The results are as follows: 35 percent of those polled thought that social stigma is "the most serious problem" facing kinky people; 54 percent thought social stigma was "a problem." Secondly, 27 percent of participants thought that isolation and difficulty in finding other kinky people is "the most serious problem," while 43 percent thought this was "a problem." The other eight issues (in order) were (3) unsafe BDSM practices, (4) sexually transmitted diseases, (5) lack of understanding between groups, (6) police harassment, (7) lack of organization/solidarity, (8) job discrimination, (9) loss of child custody, and (10) loss of leather heritage.


## FOUR KINKY TYPES TO WATCH OUT FOR

I've been so nice that now, at last, I am going to show you my dark side. In "Four Kinky Types To Watch Out For," I describe a few types of people who unfailingly set my teeth on edge.

### 1. The "Insta-Pervs"!

One minute they are the nerds next door who couldn't get a date if their lives depended on it, and the next day they are "Lord Sasquatch, Royal Dominant Master of the Dark Realm."

Or they are lonely, unhappy neurotics who transform, literally overnight, into "Dark Goddess Empress Theodora." They've never dominated anyone yet they present themselves as experienced, sophisticated players, deserving of the greatest respect. You can usually tell just how dominant they are when you meet their dogs: they invariably own dogs who mess in the house and jump on visitors like they were the holiday turkey and all its trimmings.

As the old saying goes, these people are legends in their own minds. Where do they come from and when will they go away? And why do so many of them find partners? It seems that for every clueless cluck who thinks that being a dominant is merely a matter of getting the right clothes and giving yourself a hifalutin title, there is sure to be a sea of equally clueless subbies who are ready to worship them.

## 2. The Faux-Mentors

The SM/fetish communities have a fine history of mentorship. Respected, experienced masters have long taught newcomers how to be responsible and exciting partners.

This tradition was established by the Old Guard and was embraced as doctrine for many years. Mentoring still exists, but the population explosion in the SM/fetish Scenes has made mentoring relationships much harder to come by.

Sadly, a new crop of individuals has leaped into the place once reserved for respected elders. I won't call them "insta-pervs" because instead of only being into SM for a day, they've probably been doing it for at least a month or two.

I was at a club with a submissive companion some months back when we were approached by a gent who introduced himself to us as "Master Hank," even though (as we soon discovered) he had never owned a slave. He politely inquired which one of us was dominant. Never mind that my spiked heels were grinding into my submissive friend's lap, that I was flagging dominant, or that Hank had earlier watched us at a fetish boutique, where my submissive friend tried on a tutu while I coaxed him on, laughing. Master Hank didn't have a clue who was on top.

I told him I was the dominant. He then told me that he was a "D&S teacher" and he volunteered to educate me. For free! Oh, joy! I believe he even generously offered to demonstrate spanking techniques to me—with me over his lap, of course.

Perhaps he was full of good intentions. But, as we all know, those pave the road to hell.

There are true teachers in SM communities, people who have made a lifetime commitment to educating themselves first and then others. The Master Hanks of the world do little more than flatter their own egos and mislead the gullible. Well intentioned or not, they are dangerous because they try to teach others before they've educated themselves.

### 3. Ms. or Mr. Machine

He walks! He talks! He whips! He binds!

But he doesn't seem to have a clue about BDSM. Or if he has a clue, it has long since rusted inside the square box that is his head.

Look, most SMers can appreciate stoicism now and then. It can indeed be quite sexy in a dominant. But when the stoicism is coming from catatonia, it's time to be scared. There are dominants who are so insensitive to the reality of their submissives—seeing them uniquely as a set of body parts, rather than as complete individuals—that it borders on sociopathic.

An anecdote to illustrate: I was chatting with a male dominant—I'll call him Todd—about the submissive woman he was involved with. She was preparing to move in with him. He seemed very pleased about all the SM things they'd done together. "So," I asked brightly, "what's she like?"

"She does very well with nipple clips," Todd said.

"No, I mean, what's she like?"

He looked puzzled and tried again. "She took a good paddling too."

"No, no, Todd!" I said, "I mean, what is she like as a person?"

"I don't understand." He looked baffled.

"Is she smart? Friendly? Funny?" For a minute, I thought he had to be putting me on. But he wasn't.

"Hmmmm . . ." he said, pensively furrowing his brow, "I never thought about her that way."

Is it just me or is the only appropriate response to this dialogue a loud "Ack!"

Todd was having SM sex with this woman, and more than that, was about to relocate her cross-country to live with him as his permanent slave. And the only thing he thought about her was that she could take a good spanking?

ACK!!!!

By the way, there is a submissive equivalent to the mechanical dominant and, yes, you've guessed it, it's the mechanical submissive. These are people who show absolutely no response to whatever it is the dominant does to them. They could be tied to a cross and beaten like rugs. They take it all in silence, barely wincing, and then, when finally unbound, look only vaguely uneasy, as if they're having a gas cramp.

But let me be charitable: If you're into necrophilia, these zombies could be just what you're looking for.

## 4. Dogmatists

No, this isn't some kind of a canine fetish. A dogmatist is someone who has a set of beliefs that he or she insists is the "one true way." They don't let facts distract them. They are rigidly wed to their beliefs, right or wrong, and won't tolerate opposing points of view.

Most of the time, we think of political or religious zealots as dogmatists. In an SM context, dogmatists are the ones who believe that there is only one real way to do SM. They do not merely set firm rules for their submissives; dogmatists are so convinced they possess the truth that they hurt others to keep their delusions going.

Here are a few examples to illustrate:

• *The Master* . . . who tells his slaves that there is only one "right way" to serve *all* masters, and convinces them that they aren't "real" or "true" submissives if they won't passively accept everything he demands.

• *The Mistress* . . . who has bought into the fictional fantasy images of femdoms she's read about in books and magazines, and treats her submissives like dirt because she believes that this is what being a dominatrix is all about.

• *The Master* . . . who writes a handbook on submission or slavery, which he claims to be a bible on how all masters should play. There's nothing wrong with a dominant setting down his or her thoughts about an ideal SM relationship on paper, and it's great if he or she finds a submissive who is excited by these ideals. But when a dominant tries to foist his theories on you, and intimidate you into accepting his way as the only way, he is simply not playing with a full deck. Watch out for such telltale phrases as "all slaves should be shaved" or "a slave must be naked with her master at all times."

There is no single path to dominance or to submission. The only "true submissive" or "true dominant" is the one who seems true to you.

## TWENTY HIGH-CULTURE KINK CLASSICS

Pornography is not the only place you can find explicit portrayals of SM sex. As anyone who's ever watched MTV or Jerry Springer, listened to Howard Stern, or even turned on the nightly news knows, our pop culture is overflowing with references to kinky sex.

The images of kinky sex we get from our entertainment media, however, are seldom flattering. For the most part, kinky sex is linked to violence, crime, psychosis, moral degeneracy—or, as in the movie *Blue Velvet,* with all four. Not surprisingly, in news stories on TV and thrillers on the bestseller lists, kinky sex almost invariably leads to death. The moral that media transmits is simply this: kink kills. (Or at least it's very, very bad for you!)

Of course, that doesn't stop writers and filmmakers from avidly exploiting SM themes to meet the appetite for perversion in pop culture's vast global audiences. People are fascinated by images of bondage and captivity, by fetish costumes and rough sex. A constant stream of thrillers and mystery novels, true-crime books and tabloid newspapers, pulp fiction and low-budget movies dish it out in orgies of sleaze. It is little wonder that the quintessential pop-culture trash flick, *Pulp Fiction,* featured the mandatory man-in-scary-bondage scene.

There are, however, a number of works that either have attempted significant, in-depth treatments of power relationships and sadomasochistic sex or have become such cult classics that they belong on this list. Although some of these also enforce prejudices against kinky sex, each has been influential, either in artistic circles or in SM circles, and usually in both.

1. *The Avengers:* This old British detective series (made into a very boring movie) is extremely popular with kinky people because of Mrs. Peele's admirable collection of fetish clothes and plots that frequently included scenes of her in bondage.

2. *Babydoll:* Elia Kazan's shocking movie (based on a play by Tennessee Williams) is the wonderfully sordid tale of a thumb-sucking, crib-sleeping shrew who mentally torments her husband.

3. The Beauty Series: A trilogy of novels by Anne Rice (writing as A. N. Roquelaire) about an imaginary world of tormented slaves. This series has become a cult classic. The three books in this series are *The Claiming of Sleeping Beauty, Beauty's Release,* and *Beauty's Punishment.*

4. *Bitter Moon:* Director Roman Polanski frequently explores SM themes in his film dramas. In this chilling movie, starring Peter Coyote, he depicts a couple's sadomasochistic journey to annihilation.

5. *Blue Angel (Der Blaue Angel):* Cinema classic starring Marlene Dietrich as the archetypal heartless, man-eating bitch.

6. *Blue Velvet:* David Lynch's surrealistic Midwestern fantasy featuring Dennis Hopper as a gas-sucking sociopathic fetishist.

7. *Claire's Knee:* Director Eric Rohmer's gentle comedy about a man's sudden, inexplicable obsession with a young woman's knee.

8. *Cruising:* Film starring Al Pacino as an undercover cop who enters the SM gay scene to investigate murders and becomes obsessed with the lifestyle. The film's bleak portrayal of the gay SM bar scene remains controversial—but who could resist the moody Mr. Pacino in black leather? (Not I.)

9. *Exit to Eden:* Anne Rice's book about an SM vacation resort (later made into a really bad film starring Dana Delaney).

Kinky Facts, Follies, and Fun 295

10. The GOR Series: A series of sword and sorcery novels by John Norman, set on a primitive planet of masters and slaves. A cult has grown up around the GOR books: This unique SM subculture bases its philosophy and sex roles on the novels.

11. *Justine:* Perhaps the most notorious of Alphonse Marquis de Sade's works, this novel recounts the often-violent sexual misadventures of an innocent girl. Ironically, the man who gave his name to "sadism," advocated a kind of sexual violence that no sadomasochist today endorses.

12. *Maitresse:* Director Barbet Schroeder's unflinching and explicit look at the life of a professional dominatrix. Starring Gerard Depardieu. An art house favorite and minor cult classic.

13. *Mr. Benson:* This classic gay SM novel by John Preston is about a submissive who meets and is later rescued by an idealized master.

14. *9½ Weeks:* An erotic novel by Elizabeth McNeill, chronicling a kinky relationship that goes out of control (later made into a film starring Kim Basinger and Mickey Rourke).

15. *Night Porter:* Film starring Dirk Bogarde and Charlotte Rampling depicting the doomed sadomasochistic obsession between a former Nazi war criminal and the Jewish woman he once tortured.

16. *Paris Is Burning:* Fascinating and sensitive documentary about the subculture of black and Hispanic transsexuals who compete in New York City's fabled drag pageants.

17. *Personal Services:* Hilarious British biopic about Cynthia Payne, the notorious madam of an SM bawdy house.

18. *Salo:* Director Pier Pasolini's excruciatingly depraved re-creation of de Sade's *120 Days of Sodom,* set during the decline and fall of Mussolini's Italy.

19. *Story of O:* Classic novel of female sexual slavery by Pauline Reage (later made into a film starring Klaus Kinski). This book has an enormous cult of followers, some of whom take on the main characters' names and emulate their behaviors.

20. *Venus in Furs:* A novel by Leopold Sacher von Masoch (for whom "masochism" was named) describing a submissive man's quest to turn his beloved into the dominatrix of his dreams.

## GAMES KINKY LOVERS CAN PLAY

Here is a fun variation on an old favorite that can help you and your partner spice things up in bed.

# Twisted Torturous Trivia Quiz

This is a trivia game for those kinky people who pride themselves on thinking they know everything about everything.

You know you who are.

Below are fifty torturous brain-teasing trivia questions designed to make you suffer. Consensually, of course. Even the most sophisticated culture vulture will find it hard to get every one right. (And, if you do, E-mail me at brame@gloriabrame.com, because I needed help coming up with all these questions and I want to know how you got so smart.)

### THE CRUEL RULES

You can play this game all by yourself, so you can slap yourself each time you're wrong, muttering, "I knew that!" Or you can play with your lover and hope he or she is the bigger loser. Or, if you really want to be cruel, inflict this on your friends.

If you play this with a group, designate one person as the official Inquisitor and scorekeeper. Pick lots from a hat to determine the order and then have the Inquisitor go around the room, asking the trivia questions. If someone gets it right, he or she can then answer the next question, continuing until he or she is stumped. Then move to the next person and repeat.

The Inquisitor will continue to ask the question until it is answered correctly. If all the players have had a shot at it, and the correct answer still hasn't been given, the Inquisitor should move on to the next question, and repeat the process.

The winner is the person who has given the most correct answers. (So make sure someone—preferably the Inquisitor—is keeping track of correct answers on a sheet of paper.)

Naturally, since this is kinky, some punishment is due the person with the least number of correct answers. But I will leave those sordid details up to you.

Finally, unless you're a cheater, you can only play this game once. Naturally, since all is fair in D&S, should a dominant decide to bone up on the answers before playing with a submissive, well, that would just give the dominant an unfair advantage! Gee! That would be so sadistic!

## THE TWISTED TORTUROUS TRIVIA QUESTIONS

1. What film showed Cloris Leachman dressed as a dominatrix and beating Harvey Korman, her sniveling submissive sidekick?

2. What bestselling novel tells the horrifying story of a woman chained helplessly to her bed after her husband dies during bondage sex?

3. What brand of beer ran a controversial ad campaign in the '90s showing a foot fetishist licking a woman's spiky boot?

4. In what year did the delicate yet dangerous stiletto first spike its way into the painful world of ladies' shoe fashions: 1755, 1855, or 1955?

5. What famous book contains the following line: "My beloved put in his hand by the hole of the door, and my bowels were moved for him"?

6. What Hollywood femme fatale wore men's clothing on-screen and off, and was also known to be ravenously bisexual?

7. What beloved '50s comedian popularized drag queen humor on television?

8. Which famous Hollywood movie star's divorce trial revealed that he like to spank his movie star wife?

9. What musical comedy tells a romantic tale about a songstress who performed in drag as a man and the man who loved her/him?

10. Which male jazz legend (much to the surprise of his ex-wives and children) was revealed—only after death—to have been a biological female?

11. In what movie did Woody Allen pay a prostitute to tie him up?

12. What slinky English actress played the inimitable Mrs. Emma Peele in *The Avengers*?

13. What high-ranking member of the Reagan Cabinet was caught in a sex scandal involving SM and "ponygirls"?

14. What former talk show host publicly admitted that he was a foot fetishist?

15. Which British poet's posthumously published letters revealed that he fantasized about whipping girls?

16. What famous Irish author's posthumously published letters revealed that he had a fetish for soiled knickers?

17. What signer of the Declaration of Independence was a member of England's notoriously kinky "Hellfire Club"?

18. What Beat poetry great wrote a D&S-themed poem titled "Yes, Master"?

19. When was the movie *Slaves in Bondage*—about naive country girls who are lured into lives of depravity at a big-city brothel—released: in the 1930s, the 1960s, or the 1990s?

20. Who did Sharon Stone tie to a bed in *Basic Instinct*?

21. Name the three actresses who strapped Dabney Coleman into a leather bondage harness in the '80s movie hit *Nine to Five*.

22. In what famous John Wayne movie did the Duke spank spunky redhead Maureen O'Hara?

23. In what popular 1969 Western did a young Glen Campbell spank a rambunctious Kim Darby?

24. In what Elvis Presley movie did the King deliver a sound spanking to blonde bombshell Jenny Maxwell?

25. What beloved TV classic regularly showed the trouble-making wife getting spanked by her handsome foreign husband?

26. What kind of songs did newspapers claim sportscaster Marv Albert sang when he dressed up in women's lingerie: Christmas carols, Broadway show tunes, or operatic arias?

27. What's the name of the actor who played Robin Williams's neurotic gay cross-dressing lover in the American remake of *La Cage Aux Folles*?

28. In what '60s song hit did Nancy Sinatra thrill foot fetishists by threatening: "One of these days these boots are going to walk all over you"?

29. What satirical '90s magazine published a cover featuring Hillary Rodham Clinton as a leather-clad dominatrix?

30. What '50s bondage pinup queen quit the sex industry and became a born-again Christian?

31. In what paean to masochism did John Mellencamp urge his lover to "sink your teeth through my bones, baby"?

32. What brilliant '60s musical satirist, and math professor, wrote "The Masochists' Tango"?

33. Who played Marilyn Monroe's two girlfriends in the cross-dressing comedy classic *Some Like It Hot*?

34. Who played the fetish-clad Emma Peele on the big screen, in the snoozer movie version of *The Avengers*?

35. How did Wonder Woman force criminals to tell the truth?

36. In what Martin Scorcese movie does Griffin Dunne accidentally stumble upon a bondage and SM scene in a SoHo loft?

37. Long before Ru Paul, what late, great African-American entertainer did a drag act?

38. What was the reason that the two male leads in the TV sitcom *Bosom Buddies* dressed and lived as women?

39. What '80s rock band made a fortune from exhorting people to "Whip it. Whip it real good"?

40. What famous eighteenth-century French philosopher freely confessed, in his frank *Confessions,* that he enjoyed the erotic pleasures of the whip?

41. Shortly before her death, French literary genius Dominique Aury created a stir by revealing that she had once written a notorious book under a pseudonym. What was the book and the pseudonym?

42. What famous German high-fashion photographer is famous for putting his models in SM poses and settings?

43. Why did the National Endowment for the Arts yank funding from an exhibit of photos by American photographer Robert Mapplethorpe and force the exhibit to close?

44. How many pairs of shoes was Imelda Marcos reported to have in her closets when her dictator husband was ousted from power? More than 1,000; more than 10,000; or more than 20,000?

45. Which offbeat comedian periodically appeared on the David Letterman show dressed only in a diaper?

46. What well-loved American breakfast cereal was originally described as a cure for masturbation?

47. The inventor of the above breakfast cereal was also famous for a spa he founded where enemas and antimasturbatory genital punishment devices were a regular part of the health regime. What's the title of the '90s movie about this American eccentric?

48. What popular actor played the transsexual football jock in the screen version of John Irving's *The World According to Garp*?

49. Which '60s cult movie hit featured, among other things, a cross-dressed Yul Brynner and a whip-cracking Raquel Welch?

50. What hilariously bad Ed Wood movie tells the story of a man who likes to wear women's angora sweaters?

ANSWERS:
Give yourself 2 points for every correct answer.

1. *High Anxiety*, directed by Mel Brooks
2. *Gerald's Game*, by Stephen King
3. Bass Ale
4. The stiletto was invented by Roger Vivier for Christian Dior in 1955
5. The Bible (Song of Solomon 5:4)
6. Marlene Dietrich
7. Milton Berle
8. Cary Grant
9. *Victor/Victoria*, starring Julie Andrews and James Garner
10. Billy Tipton
11. Woody Allen's *Deconstructing Harry*
12. Diana Rigg
13. Alfred Bloomingdale
14. Arsenio Hall
15. Philip Larkin
16. James Joyce

17. Benjamin Franklin
18. Allen Ginsberg
19. The 1930s
20. Michael Douglas
21. Jane Fonda, Lily Tomlin, and Dolly Parton
22. *McClintock*
23. *True Grit*
24. *Blue Hawaii*
25. *I Love Lucy*
26. Broadway show tunes
27. Nathan Lane
28. "These Boots Are Made for Walking"
29. *Spy* magazine
30. Betty Page
31. "Hurts So Good"
32. Tom Lehrer
33. Jack Lemmon and Tony Curtis
34. Uma Thurman
35. By tying them with her golden lasso
36. *After Hours*
37. Flip Wilson (as "Geraldine")
38. So they could live cheaply at an all-women's hotel (but give yourself 1 point if you said "denial")
39. Devo
40. Jean-Jacques Rousseau
41. The book was *Story of O* and the pseudonym was Pauline Reage
42. Helmut Newton
43. Because some of the pictures showed explicit SM
44. More than 20,000
45. Chris Elliott
46. Kellogg's Cornflakes
47. *The Road to Wellville*, starring Anthony Hopkins
48. John Lithgow
49. *The Magic Christian*
50. *Glen or Glenda?*

## THE CRUEL SCORING GUIDE

**80–100** points means you are an unrepentant pervert who sees SM everywhere and will go anywhere to see more.

**60–80** points means you're something of a genius, but haven't made that lifetime commitment yet to destroying your morals.

**40–60** is better than average, but you need to work on your cultural perversions.

**0–40** You're living in a cultural vacuum, baby! Wake up and smell the leather!


## KINKY READING LIST

Below is a general list of nonfiction books about kinky sexuality. Most of them were written by people involved in a BDSM lifestyle, though I've included a few scholarly works to round out your education. There are many more titles available, so this list is not a complete bibliography.

*Anal Pleasure and Health* by Dr. Jack Morin. A basic guide for men and women by a doctor and personal enthusiast.

*The Art of Sensual Female Dominance* by Claudia Varrin. A longtime dominatrix shares techniques and advice.

*Beneath the Skins: The New Spirit and Politics of the Kink Community* by Ivo Dominguez, Jr. An exploration of the political and philosophic aspects of the Scene by an SM activist.

*Between the Cracks: The Daedalus Anthology of Kinky Verse,* edited by Gavin Geoffrey Dillard. A collection of poems on kinky themes, from classic poets to contemporary ones.

*Biological Exuberance: Animal Homosexuality and Natural Diversity* by Bruce Bagemihl. A groundbreaking study of sexual diversity in other species.

*Coming to Power* by Samois, edited by Pat Califia. An early, groundbreaking collection of personal and political essays about the lesbian SM experience.

*Consensual Sadomasochism* by William Henkin, Ph.D., and Sybil Holiday. A basic guide to psychological safety issues in SM by a bisexual, switch couple.

*Different Loving: The World of Sexual Dominance and Submission* by Gloria G. Brame, William D. Brame, and Jon Jacobs. A scholarly study of kinky sex, drawing on hundreds of interviews.

*Learning the Ropes* by Race Bannon. An introductory guide to safe and consensual BDSM from a gay perspective.

*Leatherfolk: Radical Sex, People, Politics,* edited by Mark Thompson. A collection of thought pieces and essays documenting the development of leather culture.

*The Leatherman's Handbook 2* by Larry Townsend. Revised edition of the first comprehensive gay male how-to guide on safe SM practices.

*Leathersex* by Joseph Bean. All about it, by prolific SM writer and director of the Leather Archives and Museum, a scholarly project in support of research on the history of the Scene.

*The Lesbian SM Safety Manual,* edited by Pat Califia. A seminal work on safety standards in SM relationships.

*The Master's Manual* by Jack Rinella and Joseph Bean. A guide to male dominance by two experienced gay leathermen.

*Miss Vera's Finishing School for Boys Who Want to Be Girls* by Veronica Vera. A book to help males bring their feminine sides to life by sex radical and former smut queen Veronica Vera.

*My Husband Wears My Clothes: Crossdressing from the Perspective of a Wife* by Peggy J. Rudd. A first-person account of the realities of being married to a transvestite.

*Myths of Gender: Biological Theories About Women and Men* by Anne Fausto-Sterling. A scholarly work by a leading sexologist.

*Screw the Roses, Send Me the Thorns* by Philip Miller and Molly Devon. A BDSM how-to guide for couples from a maledom/femsub point of view.

*Second Coming: A Leatherdyke Reader,* edited by Pat Califia and Robin Sweeney. An anthology of essays on SM by sex radicals.

*Sensual Magic* by Pat Califia. A guide to spiritual SM for couples.

*Some Women,* edited by Laura Antoniou. An anthology of writings by lesbian SMers.

*Ties That Bind* by Guy Baldwin. A psychologist and well-known Scene activist's thoughtful essays on leathersex.

*The Ultimate Guide to Anal Sex for Women* by Tristan Taormino. Information and advice on safe, pleasurable anal sex.

# APPENDIX

# Speaking the Kinky Lingo

If you explore the organized communities of SM/fetish sex, you will come across a plethora of words, acronyms, and terms that may be unfamiliar to you. This subcultural slang is used to help kinky people clarify what they do with their partners. The slang comes from all corners of the kinky world—gay, lesbian, professional domination, leather, fetish. The Internet too has given rise to a variety of terms relevant to kinky people.

Below is a primer that should cover almost all your needs in understanding what people are talking about. Some terms left off (like spanking, whipping, flogging, etc.) are plain English and do not require special definitions here.

Most of these terms are not set in stone. Indeed, people may disagree with some of my definitions. It's also important to note that the definitions of all the terms below are continually evolving, as people debate their meaning and strive to find new ways to articulate the realities of kinky sex.

Finally, please note that some activities below, especially those identified as edge-play, are frowned upon by experienced players.

## A GLOSSARY OF SCENE SLANG

*Adult Babies:* Also known as ABs or infantilists, these are people who get erotic and emotional pleasure from wearing diapers or acting like babies.

*Age-Play:* When one partner assumes the role of the adult in the relationship and the other assumes the role of the child. Age-play is usually role-play only, but some couples extend it to lifestyle and remain in role with each other at all times.

*Animal Training:* Fantasy play in which one partner is an animal trainer and the other is the animal. Pony-play and dog-play are the two most popular forms this takes. Fantasies include obe ence training, exercise training, paper training (in dog-play), harnessing and riding (in pony-play), and so on. Other popular animal roles include cats (especially kittens), tigers, pigs, cows, and worms.

*B&D:* Acronym for Bondage and Discipline, also written as BD or B/D, and sometimes combined with SM to form BDSM. B&D is an old expression and is still used fairly interchangeably with D&S and SM, but some people define B&D as bondage and discipline without pain, and also without defined power roles.

*BDSM:* This portmanteau covers most SM/fetish-related kinks. It is a popular way of linguistically uniting the various types of players whose actual practices may differ.

*Bear:* A hairy, often large-sized, and typically cigar-smoking man, usually gay. There is a subcult of kinky people who are hopelessly turned on by bears.

*Bi-Kinky:* Someone who is heterosexual when it comes to penetration but will do SM with same-sex partners

*Biological Female/Male:* Refers to someone's sex at birth. A biological female (also known as "gender girl" or "gg") was born with the sex organs of a female, and a biological male was born with male organs. (See "transgenderism," below.)

*Black Party:* A party, usually at a gay leather club, which only people dressed in black clothes (and preferably black leather) may attend.

*Blood Sports:* Radical SM play involving cutting, piercing, or anything else that deliberately draws blood.

*Body Modification:* This includes tattooing, branding, corsetting, piercing, binding or distending flesh, cutting, and any other things people do to alter their body in primitive ways.

*Body Service:* When a submissive takes care of all the dominant's bodily needs, acting as a trained servant in bathing, shaving, hairstyling, manicures, pedicures, and other hygiene and grooming rituals.

*Body Worship:* Oral service (including licking, sucking, and kissing) by a submissive to the dominant. Implies no taboos or inhibitions about oral contact with any and all body parts.

*Bootboy:* Submissive (usually gay) male who has a fetish for leather boots worn by tops, and who frequently works at a leather bar or charitable event shining shoes. The conclusion to the shoeshining often is oral service to the boots. (See "boot worship" under "foot worship," below.)

*Bottom:* Person who receives pain or bondage in an SM scene, but who may or may not have a power relationship with the top. Also used as a verb ("to bottom").

*Boy:* Widely applied to male submissives, but has special meaning in gay leather culture, where it may also refer to the submissive partner in a daddy/boy relationship. Also used in lesbian culture to denote a male-identified (but biologically female) bottom. Used with less frequency among heterosexuals (to mean the same things).

*Breath Control:* A form of edge-play in which the top restricts the bottom's ability to breathe, either by constricting the neck or by blocking the mouth or nose. It's important to point out that this is done for extremely tiny intervals, and seldom to the point of unconsciousness. This activity is controversial because it is dangerous and potentially fatal.

*Brown Showers:* Being pooped on (or doing the pooping on someone).

*Butch:* Usually refers specifically to lesbians who express a masculine identity, but can apply to any women who seem mannish. The butch is usually the top in a leather relationship.

*CBT, CBTT:* Acronyms for, respectively, "cock-and-ball torture" and "cock, ball, and tit torture." CBT refers to any sadistic play with male genitalia; tit torture means rough play with nipples (male or female).

*Collaring:* A ceremony in which a submissive formally accepts the dominant's "collar" and becomes "officially" owned. It is the BDSM equivalent of a wedding, and is witnessed by friends and other people friendly to the lifestyle.

*The Community:* A blanket term used to refer to the organized SM/fetish communities, including the thousands of leather clubs, SM venues (bars and play-spaces), educational outreach groups, social clubs, support groups, and all other organizations that openly celebrate SM/fetish sex. The Community does not include everyone who is interested in kink but is limited to those who actively seek out and maintain close social contact with other kinky people through groups and organizations.

*D&S:* Also known as dominance and submission, DS, D/S, or D/s. Sometimes called "power relationships" (see "power exchange" and "TPE," below). D&S may be used interchangeably with B&D or SM; or it may be used to refer to a power relationship, where one partner is the sexual dominant and the other is the submissive.

*Daddy:* Anyone who assumes a paternal/mentoring role with a submissive or bottom and, in that role, expresses a masculine identity. (In other words, lesbian, bi, and het women may take the daddy role with their partners if they enjoy transgender play.) Daddy/boy relationships also exist in the non-leather gay community: among non-kinky gays, daddy/boy relationships are generally focused on mentoring and caretaking.

*Dominant:* A woman or man who assumes sexual (and possibly more far-reaching) control over a submissive partner.

*Dungeon:* Any space set aside for SM activity, public or private, and furnished with some SM equipment. Not all dungeons have large-scale equipment—home dungeons, because of space limitations, may have only small toys.

*Edge-Play:* SM that is on the edge of safety. No area of SM raises more controversy, as a good number of people feel that no one should walk the edge. Others obviously disagree.

*Electro-Play/Electrotorture:* Using devices such as violet wands for stimulation.

*Fat Admirer:* Also known as FA. A person who has a fetish for fat people. A "feeder" is a dominating person who derives pleasure from watching their partners consume large quantities of food and who actively encourages (or compels) them to gain more weight. "Feeding" could be considered edge-play in that obesity causes serious health problems. There are also FAs who simply appreciate a BBW (big, beautiful woman) or a bear and who don't want power over their partner's eating habits or weight.

*Femme:* Usually refers specifically to a feminine lesbian (may also be known as a "lipstick lesbian")—i.e., one who outwardly conforms to conventional female role models but who is bisexual or lesbian. Used, but rarely, to refer to het women.

*Fisting:* Also known as fist fucking, FF, and handballing, it's the slow insertion of a hand into a vagina or anus. Some tops will ball their hands into fists once inside, depending on the receptivity of the bottom, ergo the term "fisting."

*Flag/Flagging:* Wearing color-coded bandannas (called "hankies" or "flags") in your jeans' back pocket to let others know what turns you on. The "hanky code" is a system—developed within the gay culture—where colors represent different kinks. The hanky code has been fading somewhat, but is still in use.

People also flag their top/bottom orientation with the left/right "code" or "convention." Dominants or tops flag on the left; submissives or bottoms on the right. This also applies to other SM attire (for example, a dominant always wears her whip on the left side of her belt).

Below, I've listed the most popular SM-type flags, according to color, and indicating what it means if you wear the color in the left or the right pocket.

- *Apricot:* Left: chubby-chaser or fat admirer; right: big person.
- *Black:* Left, heavy top/sadist; right: heavy bottom/masochist.
- *Black velvet:* Left, voyeur; right: exhibitionist.
- *Brown:* Left: likes to be on top for watersports ("scat" or coprophilia and also enemas); right: likes to be on bottom.
- *Charcoal:* Left: top with a latex/rubber fetish; right: bottom with a latex/rubber fetish.
- *Dark pink:* Left: likes to give nipple pain; right: likes to receive nipple pain.
- *Gray:* Left: likes to do bondage as a top; right: likes to be bound.
- *Houndstooth:* Left: likes to bite; right: likes to be bitten.
- *Lavender:* Left: likes to top cross-dressers; right: likes to wear drag.
- *Light pink:* Left: likes to use dildos on people; right: likes to have dildos used on her/him.
- *Purple:* Left: likes to pierce; right: likes to be pierced.
- *Rust:* Left: likes to play with "ponies"; right: likes to be the pony.
- *Tan:* Left: likes to smoke cigars and play with hot ash; right: wants to worship cigar smoker and receive hot ash.
- *Yellow:* Left: likes to be on top for golden shower scenes; right: likes to receive golden showers.

*Foot-Play:* Erotic interactions with feet and all forms of foot fetishism (see chapter 7 on fetishes).

*Foot Worship:* Also called "foot service." Oral service (licking, kissing, sucking) to bare feet.

*Forced Feminization:* This is when a dominatrix (or sometimes a male dominant) "forces" a submissive man into feminine clothes (see chapter 9 on transgenderism).

*French Maid:* Fantasy role-play in which the submissive (male or female) is dressed in a French maid's uniform and serves food, drinks, and so on. The uniform usually comprises a very short, one-piece dress, often made of fetish material; a frilled petticoat; a frilly apron; stockings and high heels; and other froufrou (such as a lacy headpiece, lace wrist-cuffs, and white gloves). See "sissy maid," below.

*Gender Dysphoria:* The clinical term applied to people who feel uncomfortable in their biological sex.

*Gender Fuck:* When someone emulates, or partly emulates, the opposite sex, often to shock others. By partly, I mean they may appear with one surprising element to their dress: For instance, a man otherwise dressed male who adds (fake) breasts to the combination; or a woman dressed in regular clothes who packs a large strap-on in her jeans. Gender fuck has a political element to it as it is intended to upset standard notions of gender.

*Golden Showers:* Also known as GS and piss-play. It specifically means to pee on someone or to be peed on. However, the term is used generically to describe the spectrum of urine-play, including ingestion, wetting one's pants (or ordering someone to wet theirs), and having one's bladder controlled (or doing the controlling) either through verbal commands or devices that prevent or cause urination.

*Gorean Master:* A male dominant who adopts the code and style of life as portrayed by the GOR books of John Norman.

*Head-Play:* Also known as mind-play, mind games, head games, head trips, and mind-fucking. This means any kind of psychological manipulation by the top which heightens anticipation and fear in an emotionally masochistic bottom and thus intensifies the bottom's erotic response. This includes everything from verbal abuse (see below) to complex scenarios that confuse or surprise the bottom into deeper subspace. A mind-fuck (deliberately misleading a partner into believing something horrible is about to happen) is the deepest level of this play.

*Kajira:* This fictional term for "slavegirl" derives from the GOR series, and denotes women who attempt to live by the standard set in the books.

*Kink-Friendly:* This describes someone who, while not necessarily kinky him- or herself, is nonetheless sympathetic and supportive to kinky people. A "kink-friendly therapist," for example, is someone who has a permissive view of kinky sex. "Kink-friendly" is also used to describe businesses that welcome leatherpeople as customers.

*Kink-Positive:* Something (such as a magazine article) that portrays kinky sex in a positive light, or someone (like this author) who espouses positive attitudes towards sexual diversity.

*LDR:* The acronym for "long-distance relationship." It originated on the Internet as shorthand for couples who form serious relationships with partners who live far away.

*LTR:* The acronym for "long-term relationship," another term born on the Internet.

*Leather Culture:* The united societies of men and women (largely gay and lesbian, but increasingly open to bisexuals and heterosexuals) who embrace the traditions, ethics, and pride of open involvement in the leather Scene. This may include (but isn't limited to) active participation in leather society and politics, the wearing of black leather, formation of leather "families," and attendance at competitions.

*Leather Family:* A surrogate, adults-only family comprised of lovers, friends, and sometimes mentors who share compatible sexual interests and sociopolitical goals. Leather families share deep, binding, and sometimes spiritual commitments to one another based on their joint devotion to all things leather. The famous phrase cited by lesbian SM activist and scholar Gayle Rubin sums it up best: "Leather is thicker than blood."

*Leathermen/Leatherwomen:* Long used to refer specifically to gay or lesbian leatherpeople, but now used more generally to apply to all people committed to leather culture. (Lesbian leatherwomen may also refer to themselves as leatherdykes.)

*The Lifestyle:* When used with "the," it usually refers to "the leather lifestyle," meaning people who embrace all aspects of leather culture in their dress, their sexual politics, their social commitments, their traditions, and their sex lives. "Being in the lifestyle" is not the same as "being a lifestyler," because someone "in the lifestyle" or "in the life" could be single or otherwise uninvolved in a full-time SM relationship.

*Lifestylers:* People who assume their dominant, submissive, top, or bottom roles as a way of life. Lifestyle relationships are role-based, but not role-play. Many lifestylers are not "in the lifestyle" in that they do not participate in the organized SM Scene, but instead conduct their SM relationships in private, at home. (See chapter 8, "Role-Play and Lifestyle Relationships.")

*Limits:* The basic set of physical or other limits that the bottom sets during negotiation. For example, if a bottom does not like anything more painful than erotic spanking, she may set a pain "limit" that rules out whippings and other intense stimuli. (See chapter 12 on submissives.) Dominants too have limits on how far they wish to go with a submissive. (See chapter 11 on dominants for a complete discussion of this.)

• *Hard Limits:* The maximum edge of someone's negotiated limit. In some cases, a hard limit is a personal choice; in others, it is a necessity to safeguard the submissive's health. For example, if the submissive is allergic to latex, any latex product is a "hard limit."

• *Pushing Limits:* By consent, submissives agree to let the dominant push him or her to a limit and slightly beyond. Most commonly this occurs when the submissive believes his limits stem from an irrational fear that he hopes the dominant will help him to overcome.

• *Respecting Limits:* A fundamental ethic among kinky people is to treat limits as a sacred trust and never to violate the submissive's trust by nonconsensually exceeding their limits.

• *Stretching Limits:* Many submissives want to see progress in their submission and hope to be able to engage in increasingly more intense sex. When dominants consensually "stretch" limits, they guide submissives gradually to be able to reach their goal by pushing their limits. A dominant's limits usually stretch over time too, usually as the dominant gains increasing self-confidence, experience, and skill with equipment.

*Master/Mistress:* A master is a male dominant; a mistress is a female dominant. Masters and mistresses (as opposed to tops) always have power-exchange relationships with their partners.

*Messy:* Usually used in combination with "wet" ("wet and messy"). Refers to a fetish for being covered, or having one's clothes covered, with wet, messy substances—typically mud or oil, but can also include body wastes or gooey foods (honey, chocolate syrup, ice cream, and so on). "Messy sex" means the people like to get gooey and get it on.

*Mind Games:* See "head-play."

*Munch:* This term originated on the Internet, and refers to a group lunch or brunch at a public restaurant where kinky people can make new acquaintances or socialize with old friends in a low-key, pressure-free "vanilla" setting.

*Negotiation:* The art and science of reaching a clear, consensual agreement with your adult partner about the type of relationship you will have and the kinds of kinky things you will do together. The negotiation process lasts as long as the couple needs to hammer these things out—it could be days, weeks, months, or even years. Couples also may renegotiate terms periodically as their relationship evolves and their needs change.

"Negotiating a scene" involves a much narrower type of dialogue, in which partners only decide on what they will do during a scene.

*New Guard:* A recent movement in the Scene that embraces many traditional Old Guard standards and updates them with some freer-flowing and more permissive attitudes towards role-playing, lifestyle, diversity, racial and gender equality, and pansexuality, attitudes that are more responsive to the needs of younger people entering the Scene.

*Old Guard:* The nearly mythic, exclusively gay male societies (circa 1940s–1950s) that established the rituals and mores of leather culture. The Old Guard took a highly regimented, quasi-militaristic approach to leathersex, and organized tight, profoundly loyal local clubs throughout the United States. Rituals, traditions, and protocols varied from group to group, though some standards of behavior (from displays of patriotism to the wearing of leather) became universal.

The Old Guard is frequently seen as a phenomenon of the older generation (men now in their sixties and seventies) and is thus considered, in some quarters, as outdated. At the same time, it is held in high reverence as the first organized effort to establish protocols of behavior that stressed honor, mutual respect, compassion, and commitment.

Old Guard influences remain profound within the Scene. Although leather families on the old models scarcely exist these days, most of today's SM traditions derive from the Old Guard, including everything from the superficial (leather dress and types of toys) to the philosophical (standards on what constitutes a moral SM relationship). Some people view Old Guard traditions as the only pure model for leathersex.

There are still a few Old Guard "tribes" around the globe (particularly in the United States and Europe). Some have opened their arms to embrace the new, more pansexual SM population into their ranks. Ironically, the trendiness of kinky sex has caused a resurgence of interest in Old Guard traditions as more people search for a sense of their history.

*Pain Slut:* A heavy masochist (male or female).

*Pain Threshold:* The limit at which pain ceases to be pleasure and becomes undesirable for the submissive or bottom.

*Pansexuality:* A political, philosophical, and social movement within the organized SM/fetish communities that unites kinky people across orientation lines (i.e., gay, lesbian, heterosexual, bisexual, and transgendered together). This movement is fairly young but already gaining widespread acceptance in North America, although the old traditions of gay-only or lesbian-only venues and events continue as well.

Politically speaking, pansexuality is a way of uniting disparate SM/fetish communities into a solid front that can more effectively fight for kinky civil rights and better educate the public about the diversity and consensuality of kinky sex.

A pansexual event welcomes people of all orientations. "Pansexual play" means that gay and non-gay alike may engage in some non-sexual SM acts together, particularly in group settings (for example, a lesbian or gay man may consent to spank members of the opposite sex at a party, though neither would sleep with or otherwise have a romantic relationship with them).

*Panty Training:* This is when a dominant "forces" a male submissive to wear panties and other embarrassing bits of feminine lingerie, both to cross-dress and humiliate him.

*Petticoat Training or Petticoating:* The same as panty training, but with ruffled slips.

*Percussion-Play:* An umbrella term used to describe all forms of striking. Spanking, paddling, slapping, whipping, flogging, and caning are all types of percussion-play.

*Permanent vs. Play Piercing:* A permanent piercing refers to the implantation of body jewelry (such as nipple rings). A play piercing is a form of radical SM play in which needles or other piercing implements are temporarily inserted in flesh, either as part of a ritual (sometimes spiritual) or for the erotic pleasure of the pain it brings.

*Play:* A popular term to describe kinky encounters. "Players," however, usually means lifestylers or people with Scene experience. "Heavy players" or "hard-core players" are those who prefer intense SM.

*Play-Partner:* Generally refers to anyone with whom one has BDSM encounters but more specifically implies a casual, for-kinky-sex-only friendship and not a committed, romantic relationship.

*Play-Space/Playroom:* Alternate term for a dungeon. Any space regularly used for SM scenes.

*Ponyboy/Ponygirl:* The submissive or bottom in an animal-play relationship (see above).

*Power Exchange:* The consensual transfer of power by the submissive to the dominant. The exchange takes place when the returned energy from the dominant empowers the submissive.

*Puppy:* The submissive or bottom in an animal-play relationship (see above).

*Pushy (or Greedy) Sub:* Usually used playfully in reference to a submissive who likes a lot of play, and will act naughty to get the dominant to take action. It can also be used to refer to submissives who push so hard that they turn dominants off.

*R/T:* Acronym for "real time." Again, another term that came from the Internet to distinguish "real" (in the flesh) from on-line/E-mail relationships.

*SAM:* The acronym for "smart ass masochist"; a bottom or sub-missive who likes to verbally tease and otherwise act feisty with a dominant, usually in hopes of a little extra discipline.

*SM:* Also written as S/M, S/m, and S&M. The abbreviation for sadomasochism.

*Safe, Sane, and Consensual (or Safe, Sane, and Mutually Consensual):* The fundamental ethical standard of kinky sex. It means that all activity between adults should be "safe" (no form of pain or stimulation that causes harm), "sane" (with respect for both body and mind), and "consensual" (all partners involved are adults who are able to give informed consent).

*Safe Word:* Also called stop word, stop code, safety code. This is a word or expression that partners agree upon which gives the bottom the right to stop the action. A "safe gesture" is used if the submissive or bottom is gagged or otherwise incapable of speaking.

*Sash Queen:* Someone who regularly participates in leather con-tests and wins awards. This term can be used to poke fun at someone who is considered vain or as a good-natured joke be-tween friends.

*Scat:* Also known as scat-play, refers to excrement. Poop, to put it more plainly. This may include enemas, brown showers, watching or being watched while expelling, being ordered to soil one's pants (or ordering someone), and (yes, I'm afraid so) eating poop.

I must interject a personal comment here. From time to time, people write me and criticize me for not being more open-minded about eating poop. After all, I seem perfectly comfort-able with many other extreme types of sex, including ones that make some of my poop-eating fans faint with horror. Am I se-cretly a prude after all?

I will explain. You can't eat poop without putting yourself at risk of disease. It is true that some people who do this don't get sick. Some people who step in front of speeding cars don't get run over, either.

Human feces (unlike urine) is, by its very nature, infested with bacteria. Bacteria is what breaks food down and turns it into waste in our alimentary canals. Those bacteria remain alive in our waste after our bodies eliminate it. A bacterial infection transmitted by ingesting feces can be fatal. There is no absolute way to protect yourself against getting one. It is purely luck of the draw, so to speak.

Therefore, to my mind, ingestion, while a perfectly acceptable fantasy, can never be acted out with a guarantee of safety, unlike many seemingly more dangerous types of SM.

My advice: Substitute chocolate. They don't call the anus "Hershey Highway" for nothing.

*Scene:* There are several definitions for this word. I list them in no particular order:

a. The Scene (always with a capital *S*) refers to the SM/fetish/leather worlds. To be "in the Scene" means that one participates, even if only nominally, in organized events and considers oneself a member of this subculture. To be "out in the Scene" means that you are a known player.

b. A scene (always with a lowercase *s*) refers to one's kink or fetish, as in "My scene is feet" (i.e., the person has a foot fetish).

c. A scene (also with a lowercase *s*) refers to a time-limited SM encounter; the synonym of session (see below). "I did a hot bondage scene with him."

d. To scene: Unfortunately for those of us who are sticklers on grammar, definition (c) of scene has morphed into a verb. It means "to do SM," as in "I scened with her the other day" or "I'll be scening with him next week."

*Session:* Professional dominants refer to their time with a client as a "session." The term has, however, spread out into the general community to refer to any time-limited SM encounter. ("I had a great session with her at the club last night.")

*Sharps:* Knives, razors, or any other instrument objects used (consensually) in edge-play. Obviously, these activities can be dangerous, even fatal, if you don't use exreme caution.

*Sissy:* May also be called sissy slut. Refers to a submissive male cross-dresser (or a male submissive who is panty trained even though he is not actually a transvestite). A "sissy maid" is a male, cross-dressed in a maid's uniform, who performs household duties and otherwise serves his dominant.

*Slave:* Someone who has made a commitment to surrender sexual control to a dominant. In lifestyle slavery, the slave commits to a total power exchange in which the dominant's power goes beyond the realm of sex and enters daily affairs.

*Slave Contract:* A document written cooperatively by the dominant and the submissive in which the negotiated terms of their relationship are set out in clear language. Contracts are usually term-limited: three months, six months, a year. Some couples sign permanent contracts, vowing a lifetime commitment.

*Subspace:* The euphoric, detached state that submissives experience in service to (or during a scene with) their dominant.

*Switch:* Someone who switches D&S roles. It can apply to someone who switches roles with one partner (sometimes being on top, sometimes being on bottom) or to someone who switches according to the natural dynamic between several partners (for example, someone may be exclusively dominant with one partner and exclusively submissive with a different partner). Also includes people who primarily take one role, but will switch on special occasions or with certain people only.

*TPE:* The acronym for "total power exchange," usually referring to a lifestyle relationship (see above) in which the submissive grants the dominant blanket consent to make all decisions, erotic and otherwise.

*24/7:* Refers to a lifestyle relationship in which partners are living together.

*Toilet Slave:* Someone who has a fetish for serving the dominant's toilet habits or who has a fetish for being ordered to clean or worship toilets. May also refer to someone who wishes to role-play as a toilet (see chapter 8, "Role-Play and Lifestyle Relationships").

*Top:* Person who gives pain or bondage in an SM scene, but who may or may not have a power relationship with the bottom. Also used as a verb ("to top").

*Top's Disease:* Refers to the clueless attitude some tops or dominants develop when their egos get so big that they offend and insult others. One form would be the delusion that being dominant means one has the right to command all the submissives one meets. Another is the delusion that the top is infallible.

*Toys:* Adult toys and particularly ones used for SM play (both large-scale and small equipment).

*Tranny-Chasers:* Specifically, the ardent male suitors of male-to-female cross-dressers and transsexuals. Generically, anyone with a fetish for transgenderists.

*Transgendered/Transgenderist:* Someone who either enjoys or needs to express an opposite-sex identity. Biological males who have female identities are called male-to-female (or m-t-f). Biological females who have male identities are female-to-male (or f-t-m). (See chapter 9.)

*Transvestite:* Also known as TV or cross-dresser, and sometimes abbreviated to "X-dresser" in writing. Someone (usually male) who finds emotional and/or erotic gratification wearing opposite-sex clothing.

*Transsexual:* Also known as TS. Someone who believes she or he was born in the wrong-sex body, and seeks to make physical changes.

*Vanilla:* A non-kinky person. It can apply to any heterosexual or homosexual who does not care for kinky sex. There are two differing roots for this term: Some claim it refers to the plainness of vanilla ice cream (as opposed to those who like more adventurous flavors); others believe it comes from techno-culture, where a "vanilla" PC means a very basic machine, without bells and whistles.

*Verbal Abuse:* Also known as VA, this refers to the cruel or mocking insults and threats that a sadistic top will shower on an emotionally masochistic bottom to push him or her further into subspace. It is the linguistic and emotional (as opposed to physical) version of pain-play.

*Watersports:* A general category that includes golden showers, enemas, and other erotic interactions involving body waste.

*WIITWD:* Acronym for "What It Is That We Do." This term was spawned on the Internet, where it gained popularity as the best single way to refer nonjudgmentally to the wide variety of ways people do kinky sex.

# Index